Staying Healthy

with

NEW

NATURAL EASTERN WESTERN

MEDICINE

Published by:
Elson Haas, MD
4340 Redwood Highway, A-22
San Rafael, CA 94903
ElsonHaasMD.com

Cover and Book Design—The Book Designers: Alan Hebel and Ian Koviak
Graphics, Charts, Design and Project Direction—Neil Murray
Argisle-isms provided as a courtesy by Bethany Argisle
Contributions from Cynthia Quattro, PA, LAc and Sondra Barrett, PhD

Printed in USA by CreateSpace

ISBN-13: 978-0692687802
ISBN-10: 0692687807

10 9 8 7 6 5 4 3 2 1

Integrating Natural, Eastern and Western
Approaches for Optimal Health

Staying Healthy

with

NEW

NATURAL

EASTERN

WESTERN

MEDICINE

Elson Haas, MD

ACKNOWLEDGEMENTS

Bethany Argisle—for inspiring my writing career and helping to begin the *Staying Healthy* series way back in 1979, when we met Neil Murray in Calistoga. As the "Queen of User Friendly" you incorporated many artists' work to make a visually inspiring and informative design that became our first book, *Staying Healthy with the Seasons*. It was followed 10 years later by a 1000+ page tome, *Staying Healthy with Nutrition*. And now decades later, we have collaborated again to create the third book of the trilogy, *Staying Healthy with NEW Medicine*. Thank you Bethany, for all your creative contributions—past, present and future.

Neil Murray—for this return adventure to book production through your editing, design, and graphics. Neil, I appreciate your perception, insights, and clarity; the inspiration you created for the content of *The Health Continuum* and *Causes of Disease* charts will help our readers. Also, **Cathren Murray**, thank you for your editorial review and support.

Sondra Barrett—thank you, friend and co-author of *Ultimate Immunity*, for your help as editor and researcher for *NEW Medicine*. Glad that your brain and heart are still working so well.

Cynthia Quattro—thank you for your collaboration and contribution to *NEW Medicine* as a practitioner—Acupuncturist and Physician's Assistant—and for your contribution to the Eastern Medicine section and general editorial review. You are a smart and wonderful practitioner and I offer my appreciation.

April Cooper—for your inspiration and support of my life and daily flow with creative ideas, exquisite rainbow and nutrient-rich cuisine. I especially appreciate your belief in the vision and success of my work and career.

Ernie Hubbard—for your support and editorial review and our alliance in positive work for the past decade.

Gigi Shames—positively delightful and wise acupuncturist—for your editing and input to the book.

Tara West—for your editorial review and for our two wonderful children, Orion and Ishara, who bring us great joy. Thank you.

Alan Dino Hebel and Ian Koviak—for being a great team of Book Designers.

Preventive Medical Center of Marin—for your support to be a unique and innovative clinic in our integrative healthcare delivery and the development of the *NEW Medicine* model. Our wonderful team helps my busy life work well.

CONTENTS

PREFACE

The Motivation for NEW Medicine

AS A PRACTICING PHYSICIAN for 40 years I see and know well the challenges of our current healthcare system. All of us—doctors and consumers alike—want and need to know how to take better care of ourselves to prevent both acute illnesses and long-term chronic conditions that too often arise later in life. This is the best Medicine! To accomplish these goals we must become better informed as patients, doctors, and medical personnel so that we know how to navigate the potentially treacherous waters of current medical choices.

Over the course of my career, my focus has been to share with others what I have learned in my practice with thousands of patients, and in my own life and health studies. This has led to many published books, articles, and presentations—embracing the original meaning of the word "doctor," which comes from the Latin for "teacher." I strive to both inform and provide practical approaches to guide people in becoming their own best doctors by preventing illness in the first place, and caring better for themselves, their families and friends, all while honoring Mother Earth.

After my medical school education and training I had an epiphany, realizing that what I had been taught equipped me to focus on illnesses and disease, but not on fundamental health and wellness. In short, I had been trained as a "symptom fixer" and "disease fighter," and not as an educator or healer. In response to this realization, I began studying and practicing a variety of alternative healing approaches that were not part of conventional Western medicine at that time. My explorations included Traditional Chinese Medicine, Naturopathy, Herbal Medicine, and Mind/Body Healing. These therapeutic modalities have become the foundation of what I call NEW Medicine—an integrative approach that incorporates the best of **"NEW"—Natural, Eastern, and Western**—approaches to optimal health.

Fortunately in these last few decades, we have seen greater acceptance of these multidisciplinary practices by Western medicine, insurance companies, and also by the general public. Many in the mainstream medical establishment now embrace this new field, which includes Complementary-Alternative-Holistic-Integrative Medicine.

Today, many medical doctors see and believe what early explorers, such as Andy Weil, Bernie Siegel, Marty Rossman, Bernard Jensen, Michael Tierra, and myself were discovering and sharing. Integrative MDs and DOs (Osteopaths) are now found in most major urban centers as are other naturally-oriented health practitioners, such as chiropractors, acupuncturists, and naturopaths who can assist and empower us to restore our health with lifestyle guidance and natural remedies and treatments.

There are also numerous educational groups and online resources training practitioners in these areas, including the Institute for Functional Medicine (IFM), American Board of Integrative Holistic Medicine (ABIHM), and the Orthomolecular Health Medicine Society (OHM). I am proud to be part of this field as a pioneer and contributor and believe that my career of practice, writing, and teaching has played some role in its evolution.

As I continue to evolve in my profession and learn and grow personally, I realize that the best way to Stay Healthy is by living true to our own guidance and mission first and foremost, and then by addressing the causes of illness, if and when they appear. To mainstream medicine, prevention mainly involves immunizations and early detection screening tests like mammograms and colonoscopies. To me, the true meaning of "Preventive Medicine" embodies the philosophy that **our Lifestyle is at the very core of our health and wellbeing,** and our daily choices often make the difference between living with chronic diseases, or experiencing vibrancy, energy, creativity and vitality.

This is often easier to talk or write about than it is to put into practice, especially with today's stress-filled, fast-paced lives, and the ready accessibility of many pre-packaged and processed "junk" foods versus natural, fresh, and organic vegetables, fruits, grains, etc. In addition, family patterns and TV advertisements often promote unhealthy habits in our young people—from what they eat and their emotional behavior, to spending too much time in front of "screens" and too little exercising and being in nature.

"Without Nature, there is no Healing."   —ARGISLE

The health of our young people is particularly important because bad habits learned early can have disastrous short-term and long-term consequences, as we see with the alarming rates of childhood obesity and early onset diabetes. Therefore a key passion throughout my career has been to reach young people with the message of *caring for the one and only body they each possess, with love and respect.* I continue to be active in teaching children about how their bodies work and how to take care of themselves by making nourishing choices and learning the difference between real food and treats. I believe that this is critically important work for each of us as individuals and as a society.

In spite of significant progress, much still needs to be done. If our current medical system is failing us, let's not first look at the politicians and policy makers. Instead, let's gaze into the mirror and ask what *we* are doing to avert and address both short-term illnesses and long-term diseases. There is so much each of us can do to maintain and even improve our health. I have put many of these principles into practice in my own life, with my family, friends, and patients in my community.

To me, the heart of a true renaissance in our healthcare system is to empower each individual with the knowledge and resources they need to make the best choices for health on a daily basis.

This book completes my **"Staying Healthy" Trilogy** that began with *Staying Healthy with the Seasons* and continued with *Staying Healthy with Nutrition.* It is about the quality of life and the quality of care that you create with your chosen doctors and health providers, so that we can all share a healthier world.

I embrace the philosopher-physician role of the Barefoot Doctors of ancient China who were primarily paid to keep people well. They were also thought to be knowledgeable about how to live life in a way that flows harmoniously with both the local environment and the grand universe.

I am excited to provide you with this new work. I believe it can empower you to create positive changes in your life so you can enjoy all of your years on our planet.

Stay Healthy!
Dr. Elson Haas
April, 2016
Sebastopol, CA

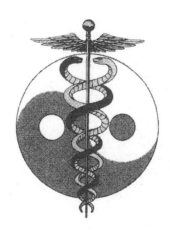

INTRODUCTION

The Current US Healthcare Crisis and a New, Practical Approach

"Wise people should realize that health is their most valuable possession."

—HIPPOCRATES

FEW WOULD ARGUE that our health—as individuals and as a society—is our greatest asset. I am talking about *physical, mental, emotional, environmental, and spiritual wellbeing and vitality,* as true health involves all of these dimensions. Without good health we may suffer and deteriorate; with it we can create, achieve and thrive.

Unfortunately the present system of health care in the US does not always serve us well (other than for crisis care), and at times it can even undermine our wellbeing. What does it say about our great nation that in spite of the good intentions of many, our political and personal priorities do not fully reflect the fact that our health is where our nation's real wealth lies?

I am fully aware and appreciative of the many great contributions made by Western medicine to the health of our nation and the world. In fact, I am in awe of the unprecedented advances in our ability to prevent and diagnose illness and to counteract most infectious diseases that devastated populations only decades ago. Improved hygiene, clean water and uncontaminated food have led to increased life expectancy over the last century. Countless lives have been saved by the judicious administration of immunizations, modern pharmaceuticals, especially antibiotics, as well as surgery and trauma care. When any of us gets acutely ill, or if we are injured in an accident, we are fortunate that we live in these modern times where Western Medicine can help us mend, recover, and return to our healthy and productive lives.

Yet, in spite of these and countless other advances, we have clearly lost our way in terms of keeping our people healthy and providing natural and preventive solutions as part of an overall healthcare system for all of our citizens.

- Should we be focusing the vast majority of our finances and research efforts on technology and drug development with virtually nothing by comparison spent on preventive and natural care?

- Should we be encouraging the consumption of unhealthy foods, beverages and drugs (by industry and advertising) instead of educating all of our citizens—young and old alike—about the importance of healthy diet, exercise, and stress reduction?

- How effective can we be in the face of an unhealthy environment?

- Why are there so many people with less than optimal health?

- Why are so many of us obese and overweight?

- Why are cancer and heart disease problems still so prevalent?

- And of equal importance in assessing the value of Western Medicine in the US, why are there still so many of us who struggle to afford basic, good quality care (even though this has improved recently)?

- How can we incentivize health-focused programs so that people will be motivated to assume responsibility and participate in their own health?

This book addresses these questions and presents an alternative vision for health care based on my 40 years as both a student of healing, and as a practicing physician. It offers practical ways that we, as individuals and communities, can meet the challenges of transforming our personal health and in the long run, that of our society as a whole.

CHRONIC DISEASE IN THE US

A significant concern within our Healthcare System (HCS) is the high incidence and cost of Chronic Diseases—namely **Cardiovascular Disease, Cancer and Diabetes**. (Note that Obesity is often an underlying factor is these three life-threatening diseases.) Our current system is partly a victim of its own success with respect to these chronic diseases. Advances in diagnosis and treatment of heart disease, stroke and cancer have resulted in fewer people dying of these illnesses. US life expectancy now averages 78.8 years—the highest in our history. The result is a rapid increase in the number of Americans who are living with chronic illnesses rather than dying from them, and this means a lot of our resources and healthcare dollars go to elder care. We now face a HCS that excels at saving lives, but is not necessarily designed to promote health or address the quality of life and the affordability of care, for people with long-term illnesses. On a positive note, no area better illustrates how our individual lifestyle choices might effect positive change **through prevention**, while improving outcomes with lower costs over time. I address this topic in more detail in *Appendix 1*.

HEALTH CARE IN THE US

In America, our health outcomes are unrewarding or mediocre at best. This includes life expectancy, infant mortality, and incidences of both chronic disease and obesity. In addition, the financial ramifications are currently beyond control for many of us and could spiral into an even greater crisis for present and future generations.[1] Unless we make the necessary changes to achieve improved health outcomes at a reasonable cost, we risk stressing our country's finances even more, especially with so many baby boomers joining Medicare currently and over the coming years.

In spite of unprecedented advances in Western Medicine over the past 50-100 years, our status in the world as a healthy nation is not what we would expect.

- The US is not one of the 10 healthiest countries in the world.[2]

- Among the wealthy countries in the world the US healthcare ranks last.[3]

- According to a 2015 international study,[4] the US ranks 34th in general thealth, below Morocco and just above Slovenia and Cuba.

The trend is clear across multiple studies comparing overall health costs and outcomes between different countries around the world; our current healthcare system is not doing a good job for our people. In the absence of a viable solution to this crisis, our present and future generations face daunting challenges to their health and in their ability to pay for essential care.

Currently, the US spends more of its wealth on health care than any other industrialized economy, yet the outcomes and benefits don't reflect these greater expenditures. Given our large national investment in this area, our citizens should be the healthiest, most vital, and longest living people on the planet, and yet we fall far short of this mark. In reality, there is a demonstrable failure of our health-care system to generate the kind of returns for its citizens that are already being enjoyed by many other countries around the world.

PER CAPITA HEALTH CARE SPENDING 2013

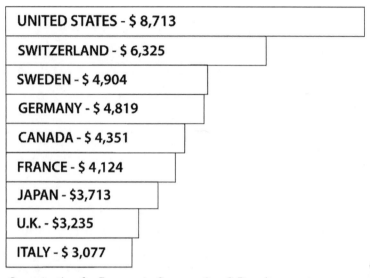

UNITED STATES - $ 8,713

SWITZERLAND - $ 6,325

SWEDEN - $ 4,904

GERMANY - $ 4,819

CANADA - $ 4,351

FRANCE - $ 4,124

JAPAN - $3,713

U.K. - $3,235

ITALY - $ 3,077

Organization for Economic Cooperation & Development
2015 Report

Ongoing attempts to reform health care through legislation have shown the difficulty of making any significant changes due to our often polarized and contentious political system. The Affordable Care Act (which I discuss in more detail shortly) has brought about some progress in this area. In addition to expanding insurance coverage Obamacare sought to lower some of the exorbitant expenses of US healthcare. Although costs have continued to rise since the passage of the bill, the rate of increase has slowed in the past few years. (In 2007, the rate was 12% and is now predicted to be 6.5% in 2016.[5]) This reverses a long-term trend and projections for the future are not as dire as they were just a few years ago.

Of course, a slowing in the rate of growth is not the same as an actual decrease and it seems clear that predicting healthcare cost trends is extremely challenging, especially with the unknown consequences of the baby boomer's aging. And we are still spending twice, and in some cases three and four times as much, as other advanced countries.

Along with political deadlock we must add the powerful influence of thousands of well-funded lobbyists representing the vested interests of the various power players such as Big Pharma and agri-business, whose agenda is often at odds with what is best for our overall health as individuals and as a society. It is clear that if we wait for change from the TOP DOWN it will be a long time, if ever, before we see any real progress. The alternative is a BOTTOM-UP, grass roots effort that begins with each of us becoming our own best primary healthcare provider, supported by positive and balanced relationships with trusted health practitioners. The key to improving our health lies much more in our own hands than we realize—and it is time to take action.

What we lack is a clear roadmap to guide us through the complexities and limitations of the current medical system toward a truly meaningful use of preventive and integrative approaches that can result in optimal health and wellness. ***Staying Healthy with NEW Medicine* is that roadmap.**

HOW DID WE GET HERE?

The crisis in our nation's health care is not new. It did not appear on the scene overnight, nor am I the first to call for change. But watching this ever-increasing decades-long crisis, I have seen the growing need for a new vision for our Healthcare System, and I have discovered, developed and applied promising key elements of that vision in my practice, with my patients and as a patient myself, and in my books and articles.

Clearly, this is a highly complex topic with economic and political ramifications beyond the scope of this book and my areas of expertise. However, I have worked as a physician within the system for many decades and can offer some basic observations about the problems and potential solutions that I see and experience both personally and professionally.

The evolution of US Health Care has been shaped by a complex spectrum of positive and negative factors, including:

- Scientific discoveries and technological advances with a focus on a Western Medical approach

- The conflict of social, political, and economic agendas, such as the promotion of unhealthy products, like tobacco, fast foods, meats, and processed sugar products, as well as GMO foods

- Insurance companies, rather than doctors, often deciding on the type and quality of care, and what is covered—primarily accepted pharmaceutical and surgical treatments.

- The significant percentage of healthcare costs resulting from chronic diseases such as cardiovascular disease, diabetes and cancer when many of these conditions can be mitigated, if not prevented, by less expensive lifestyle-based treatments.

- The disproportionate amount of our healthcare dollars spent on end-of-life medical care, especially in hospitals and ICU's.

The end result is that we do not actually have a healthcare system in the US. What we have is a DISEASE CARE SYSTEM. The focus is more on doing tests, performing procedures, prescribing drugs, treating symptoms, and attempting to manage chronic health problems rather than achieving optimal health through education, healthy lifestyles, and natural preventive care. Also our current HCS is not really a "system" at all, but rather a dysfunctional hodge-podge of institutions and disease treatments that has evolved over the last century.

THE OTHER PATIENT—THE SYSTEM

Treating thousands of people over the years, I have come to realize that the real patient isn't only the person in my reception room, or on my exam table. The doctor's office is extremely crowded with many of the invisible participants in the HCS: the government, the patient's insurance company, the legal system, and the pharmaceutical industry to name just a few—they are all present and often part of the problem and in need of treatment!

This complex and dysfunctional system has evolved since the Industrial Revolution in the West, with its myopic focus on modern technology and short-term solutions, its heroic attitude of "crisis care," and ultimately its emphasis on profit above all else. **This focus has led us away from a fully integrated approach that ideally addresses and corrects the underlying causes of ill health and disease. It's a system that has disconnected us from Nature, which is in fact one of the most important guides to true and lasting health.**

Since my graduation from medical school in 1972, I have witnessed an ever-increasing power alliance between major factions and sectors in our medically-oriented society. The following chart represents the many players involved in our HCS. YOU are in the middle of all of this! See yourself in the chart.

THE COMPLEXITIES OF OUR CURRENT HEALTHCARE SYSTEM

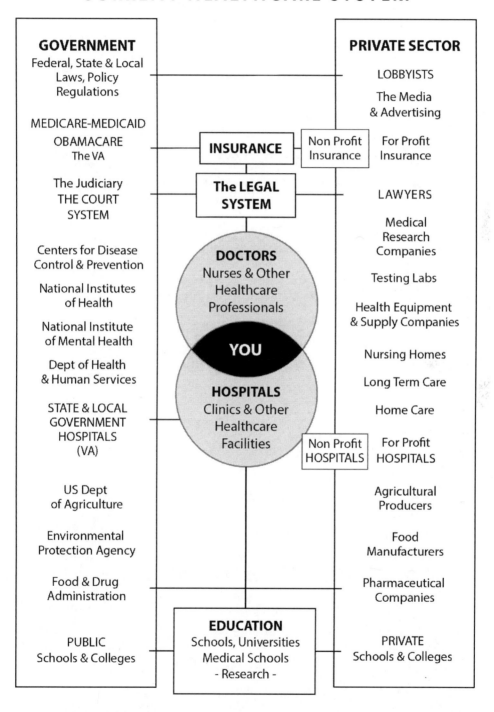

GOVERNMENT
Federal, State & Local
Laws, Policy
Regulations

MEDICARE-MEDICAID
OBAMACARE
The VA

The Judiciary
THE COURT
SYSTEM

Centers for Disease
Control & Prevention

National Institutes
of Health

National Institute
of Mental Health

Dept of Health
& Human Services

STATE & LOCAL
GOVERNMENT
HOSPITALS
(VA)

US Dept
of Agriculture

Environmental
Protection Agency

Food & Drug
Administration

PUBLIC
Schools & Colleges

PRIVATE SECTOR
LOBBYISTS

The Media
& Advertising

Non Profit Insurance | For Profit Insurance

LAWYERS

Medical
Research
Companies

Testing Labs

Health Equipment
& Supply Companies

Nursing Homes

Long Term Care

Home Care

Non Profit HOSPITALS | For Profit HOSPITALS

Agricultural
Producers

Food
Manufacturers

Pharmaceutical
Companies

PRIVATE
Schools & Colleges

INSURANCE

The LEGAL SYSTEM

DOCTORS
Nurses & Other
Healthcare
Professionals

YOU

HOSPITALS
Clinics & Other
Healthcare
Facilities

EDUCATION
Schools, Universities
Medical Schools
- Research -

WHERE DOES THE MONEY GO?

Given the significant focus on the profit motive[6] within our health-care system and related industries, it is no wonder that previous attempts at reform have been largely unsuccessful. To put it bluntly, there are literally too many factions fighting for the money, and too little regard for long-term health outcomes and costs to patients and the HCS in general.

Currently preventive care in our country is not big business, especially compared with the many powerful players in today's HCS who may be valuing money over true health. Our present system is driven by expensive lab tests, x-rays, CAT scans, and MRI's, various procedures, and especially prescription medicines. So it is not surprising that this is where most of the money is made—by hospitals, drug companies, insurance companies, medical equipment manufacturers, labs, clinics and practitioners recommending, conducting and analyzing diagnostic tests. Many of these companies continue to make obscene profits. We can change our needs for their use with more informed decisions and better personal health. Let's now look at some examples of the many participants of our HCS.

HOSPITAL AND EMERGENCY ROOM CARE

Key contributors to healthcare costs are the exorbitant prices that hospitals and emergency rooms can charge. These are highlighted in Steven Brill's book *America's Bitter Pill*[7] in which he gives multiple examples of the "Chargemaster" schedules held by most hospitals, with costs that are often 10–100 times more per pill, medical supply, procedure, or service provided than would typically be covered and paid by Medicare and insurance companies. For example:

$1.50 for one acetaminophen pill (generic Tylenol)—at the time you could buy 100 of them on Amazon for $1.49.

$283 for a simple chest X-ray, for which the hospital in question was routinely paid $20.44 by Medicare.[8]

$13,702 for an injection of a cancer drug when the average price paid by all hospitals for this drug was $4,000.

The chart below shows a similar example from my own experience. These numbers are from a bill given to me by a patient for his ER visit several years ago. I find the amounts that the hospital billed the insurance company unfathomable. I still see this kind of issue consistently.

TEST	Hospital	My Clinic or Typical Coverage
Complete Blood Count	$482	$15–$30
Comprehensive Metabolic Panel*	$710	$40–$60
EKG Electrocardiogram	$617	$45–$75
TOTAL	**$1809**	**$100–$165**

a panel of 10-15 tests like blood sugar, sodium, kidney and liver function

If someone has insurance, neither the patient nor the insurance company would likely pay that much; yet, the private-pay or uninsured patient might be stuck with these charges. This bill is ill! It is suffering from a serious case of obesity! It's sad to see that such practices have caused many people to lose everything—their homes, savings, relationships, and even their health.

PHARMACEUTICAL COMPANIES

I am both impressed and depressed with the ever-increasing power of the pharmaceutical industry—the ultimate "symptom fixer." In many respects, we have become a "drug culture," both in lifestyle and in our approach to dealing with health issues. Making symptoms disappear temporarily without addressing the underlying cause is not the answer. If addressing fundamental health issues truly mattered to our policy makers and businesses, there would clearly be a much greater emphasis upon lifestyle and other natural, preventive approaches to dealing with underlying causes of poor health. Unfortunately, research on lifestyle is expensive and demanding, requiring decades of follow-up. It is much easier to follow the test results of drugs targeted against specific illnesses often supported by the drug companies themselves, that also support research at medical schools. We clearly have a drug-pushing approach in our healthcare system. For example:

> Percent of physician office visits involving drug therapy: 75%
>
> Percent of persons using at least 1 prescription drug in the past 30 days: 49%
>
> Percent of persons using 3 or more prescription drugs in the past 30 days: 22%[9]

Big Pharma markets directly to doctors with all kinds of promotions, millions spent in medical journal advertising, and many freebies and perks besides free samples. It's not just about profits. In the US there is no government regulation of prices as there is in other countries.[10] Why do drugs cost so much in the US when the same drugs can be found for much less in most other countries? This situation drives many people to buy their prescription medicines in such places as Canada, Mexico, and India.[11]

There are also many "downstream" pollution effects resulting from our disposal of medicines. This especially creates contamination in our water supplies and the Earth's waterways.

80% of the US's streams and nearly a quarter of the nation's ground-
water sampled by the United States Geological Survey has been found
to be contaminated with a variety of medications.[12]

DRUG ADVERTISING

Perhaps a good start in decreasing drug costs would be to eliminate
television advertising for drugs as we did for tobacco. The sales and
profits of the drug companies have been greatly enhanced by aggres-
sive direct to consumer advertising (DTCA) campaigns in print
and on television. The only other developed country to allow such
advertising for pharmaceutical drugs is New Zealand. We have all
witnessed the results in the proliferation of drug commercials, often
with lengthy side effect statements. Despite the fact that pharmaceutical companies often justify their profits as necessary to fund
research and offset risk, they typically spend significantly more on
marketing and promotion than on Research & Development.

Drug DCTA has been legal in the USA since 1985, but only really took
off in 1997 when the FDA eased up on a rule obliging companies to
offer a detailed list of side effects in their infomercials. Since then the
industry has poured money into this form of promotion with expenditures rising from $1.1 billion in 1998 to $4.5 billion in 2014.[13]

**On November 17, 2015, in response this situation, The
American Medical Association called for a ban on direct-
to-consumer ads for prescription drugs and implantable
medical devices, saying they contribute to rising costs
and patients' demands for inappropriate treatment.**

AGRIBUSINESS

Even with the significant growth in organic farming and natural food store sales, we have still taken a similar approach to farming that we have to medicine—an "attack and conquer" mentality that identifies an "enemy"—in this case insects, pests and weeds—and then eradicates them with strong chemicals to help farmers supposedly grow their crops better. Raising livestock or poultry with the use of antibiotics and growth hormones raises similar issues. We also want to protect our waters, earth, air and those who work the land, from contamination. Of course, costly agricultural chemicals may help farmers produce their crops more efficiently and profitably, yet the chemicals have depleted the soil and contaminated our food and the environment. Surely we must realize that what we do to the land—the Earth—we eventually do to ourselves as these chemicals get into our bodies where they can negatively impact our health. Studies by the CDC have revealed up to 265 man-made chemicals in human tissue samples.[14]

FOOD MANUFACTURING

Good nutrition is a foundation of health, so the quality of our food supply is critical. We are always going to be exposed to a wide variety of chemicals, yet whatever we can do to lessen and limit this overall exposure is essential. We can accomplish this by using fewer toxic chemical products where we can at home, at work and on our body. The use of GMO foods, sometimes called "Frankenfoods," is another part of this profit-focused, product development world. Even with the potential they offer for growing more food, Genetically-Modified Organisms represent a mass human experiment, what some have even called "genetic roulette." And what about the bees and other pollinators? Their numbers have declined dramatically over the past few decades with the increased use of toxic environmental chemicals and GMO plantings.

Like the pharmaceutical industry, the big business of food production employs well funded and highly sophisticated marketing tactics—much of it targeted at our nation's young—that would have us believe in the benefits of many processed products that typically contain lots of fat, too many calories, chemicals, potentially harmful additives and no real nutritional value. This pertains largely to packaged foods, sugary cereals, candy, sodas and unhealthy fast foods, often promoted by sports heroes or movie stars. Besides the ill effects on consumers, this creates a major challenge for health practitioners working with nutrition and lifestyle.

MEDICAL EQUIPMENT AND SUPPLIES

Our current medical culture has created an unceasing demand for the latest and greatest technical discoveries. Why? One reason is that they bring in ever-increasing revenues and profits. Medical equipment and supply companies rank with drug companies as among the most profitable in the country.[15] Of course, they also help us diagnose medical problems. Still, in a vast majority of tests, findings fall into the normal range, so that makes us wonder if they are all needed, or can improved screening (taking better histories and more thorough exams) save money with more accurate clinical assessments and less testing?

Experts say that spending on new health technology—not only sophisticated machines, but also new specialty drugs, devices, procedures, and cyber security—continues to add to the annual increases in healthcare costs.[16] It's one of the key reasons why US healthcare is so expensive. The problem isn't usually the technology itself, but rather its over-use in certain situations where it hasn't been shown to help more than cheaper options. This might include CT scans for many patients who come into the ER with conditions such as abdominal pain, back pain, or headaches. Because the technology is available, it is often recommended and it protects the hospitals and doctors from a missed diagnosis, and of course, it provides significant revenue.

Beyond the actual necessity of a new device or test, our system ingrains the notion that people deserve—and will benefit from—the newest test, procedure, or treatment. This progressive focus on invention and discovery has certainly helped advance our medical system, yet it adds competition and cost to our HCS without necessarily improving real health outcomes. Of course, some may be great breakthroughs in medical technology and can help many patients, but we need to be more discriminating about the real health benefits of innovation.

> In a study of more than a million Medicare patients, researchers looked at how often people received one of 26 tests or treatments that scientific and professional organizations have consistently determined to have no benefit or to be outright harmful. They reported that in a single year, 25% to 42% of Medicare patients had received at least one of the 26 useless tests and treatments.[17]

HEALTH INSURANCE

This complex sector of our HCS affects how we protect and support our population to provide quality medical care at affordable prices, but the situation is clearly out of hand with premiums and deductibles increasing every year. The Affordable Care Act does not seem to have changed the situation appreciably. The legislation mainly improves access to healthcare by subsidizing coverage for people of lower income rather than improving health care itself.

THE AFFORDABLE CARE ACT (ACA)

Here are some thoughts on "Obamacare," from a practitioner's viewpoint. Let's be clear about this: It is not really about health care reform;[18] it is an improved insurance program with greater accessibility to coverage and subsidies going to people of lower income to help them, even require them, to have coverage. Thus, it provides some basic services at a relatively low price to those in need, and more adults and children have insurance coverage, and that's great. I am seeing people for check-ups who have not used the system for exams and blood tests in many years. From my perspective, this is the strength of the ACA. Also, it does support the yearly "preventive medicine or health evaluation" and requires that insurance companies offer this "well-check," when not all of them did before. Furthermore, it doesn't allow insurance companies to use pre-existing diagnoses and conditions to deny coverage.

What's the cost? Plenty is the simple answer. First of all, many who do not qualify for subsidies based on low income are paying much more—double in many cases—and that's for less coverage, with higher deductibles and greater co-pays. So they are getting less for more, whereas those that qualify are getting more for less. In my view, the insurance companies are the big winners here, and the government is spending our tax money to fund this program. This is different from Medicare, where people have paid into Social Security over many years to qualify for their benefits. In my opinion, we can do even more to provide better care to our citizens.

If this trend of increasing insurance prices continues, we will eventually bear a greater and greater burden of financing our own health care and the government and tax payers will be covering the cost of ACA subsidies. Ironically, this trend may lead us—of necessity—to a more preventive, integrative and cost effective approach, but why should this have to occur as a consequence and not as a logical approach to the dilemma we face?

Ideally, in addition to having insurance, we should first have **Health Assurance**—*knowing how we can live our lives in ways that foster our health, and that we are sharing this knowledge and experience with our families and friends.*

THE LEGAL SYSTEM

Issues surrounding medical malpractice and the fear of malpractice lawsuits definitely affect the quality and cost of medical care. This area of our HCS is extremely complex, with many financial and ethical dimensions, and it needs a comprehensive and innovative solution that protects all parties involved. When doctors and hospitals practice defensively to avoid lawsuits, they tend to order more potentially unnecessary tests in order to make sure they don't miss a diagnosis. A missed diagnosis is one of the most frequent types of medical malpractice lawsuits, leading to a growing trend on the part of doctors to make sure their records indicate they did everything possible to test the patient. Not only does this place legal protection above true patient care, the cost of testing in our county is another reason why medical costs have skyrocketed.

According to recent surveys,[19] physicians estimate that defensive medicine practices cost the US between $650 and $850 billion annually. Physicians attributed 34% of overall healthcare costs to defensive medicine and 21% of their practice to be defensive in nature. Specifically, they estimated that 35% of diagnostic tests, 29% of lab tests, 19% of hospitalizations, 14% of prescriptions, and 8% of surgeries were performed to avoid lawsuits.

HEALTHCARE: A HUMAN RIGHT?

Finally, why is the US the only advanced country where access to affordable health care is not viewed as a basic universal right, like the education of our young people? Obamacare just begins to address this issue. When it comes to universal health care, the United States is the lone exception among developed nations. Such coverage does not necessarily imply a government-only solution, since many countries with such plans have a two-tier system with both public and private insurance and medical providers.

Will there come a day where excessive profits from human disease and suffering will seem as unacceptable as war profiteering? We can create a system that addresses our people's health needs, offers every person working in the HCS fair compensation for their work, training and expertise, yet does not charge excessively to pad the pockets of the many invested parties that play a role in our healthcare system?

WHAT WE NEED NOW

This book addresses the many things we can do to improve our personal health and our HCS. In my view, there are new responsibilities that need to be adopted by patients, practitioners, hospitals, and by our entire national healthcare system.

OUR ROLE AS PATIENTS

The origin of some of our HCS dilemmas also lies in the fact that as patients and consumers, we have basically accepted the system of "quick fixes" with drug therapies and the latest, greatest tests and treatments, including organ and body part replacements and cosmetic enhancement surgeries. Most of these "advances in Western Medicine" are oriented toward eliminating or minimizing negative symptoms, not preventing them in the first place through incentives and proactive lifestyle education. Really, there should be no greater incentive than our own health and vitality. Many of us have never learned how to care properly for our own bodies and minds, and we assume that when things go wrong with our bodies, our doctors will fix us. **Furthermore, many of us race toward Western technological medicine as the ultimate answer to nearly all of our health care needs, and we have—in the process—played our part in creating a system that is itself in need of healing.**

PERSONAL ACCOUNTABILITY

In addition, our current HCS often ignores personal accountability for our own health, and many people assume that the medical establishment (with urgent and emergency care, hospitals and pharmacies) can save them regardless of how they care (or don't care) for themselves. Of course, this pervasive view leads to a self-perpetuating crisis, since many people with unhealthy lifestyles and habits won't enter the system until they need rescuing with costly interventions, and might even be beyond any hope of real recovery or cure.

Often people don't seek care because they can't afford it. This has improved somewhat with the Affordable Care Act and more people having insurance coverage. Still, this "waiting for a crisis" before seeking care gives rise to at least two other problems—more visits to expensive emergency rooms, urgent care facilities and intensive care units; seeking the least expensive care due to the high cost of co-pays or deductibles; and in some cases, seeking no care at all, even when it would be beneficial. We need to reach out and educate our society (and politicians) to make individual accountability a key part of our future HCS with a more equitable, affordable insurance system. When people realize that their health is their most valuable possession and that feeling good, even great, is its own reward, they can be motivated to be proactive in protecting and supporting their own health. This can lead to lower costs for individuals, insurance, and for our system as a whole.

A GREATER FOCUS ON PREVENTIVE CARE

Within the current system, there are minimal financial incentives for providing basic, preventive patient care. Such care is often relatively time-consuming and typically not covered fully by insurance, or when it is covered only a minimal and insufficient amount of time is allowed. This has improved in recent years with progressive business programs as well as more insurance companies offering or paying for annual health exams and visits. Yet, more is needed as a society to create greater incentives for doctors and their medical staff to offer these crucial preventive services, such as nutritional counseling, weight loss and stress management, which ideally should be insured and reimbursed at better rates. This includes taking more time educating patients, especially in helping them change their long-term lifestyle patterns rather than simply relying on quick reviews and temporary treatments.

Unfortunately the way our current HCS is structured, with much greater compensation to specialists and urgent/emergency care, it's fairly obvious why the number of general and family practitioners is declining, yet these are the very doctors we need most to provide education and motivation about prevention. We can remedy this when the government aligns with the medical schools and societies to set up better incentive packages to encourage the family doctor.[20]

NEW SOLUTIONS: WHAT CAN WE DO?

Although this book covers a wide range of topics, I am focusing on **two key approaches—personal responsibility and widespread public education**—to bring sustainable health to all of us. Working within an integrative medical model at my clinic and using insurance (mostly a fee-for-service system), I have directly experienced that we can often get better results with less expense. As suggested already, this can occur most readily when the patient and doctor work cooperatively to look at causes, often lifestyle-based, and take steps to undo the disease patterns and move toward enhanced health activities. This is most effective when we focus on prevention early in the process. For example, by doing a better job managing people with elevated blood pressure, cholesterol, or blood sugar levels—these early chronic diseases, which can become extremely expensive over time, but can also be reversed, or at least delayed by years, through lifestyle changes. Such steps can make a significant reduction in costs and improvement in health. Of course, this will be better facilitated when we build in those incentives for "good behavior" just as good drivers pay less for their auto insurance, or people who don't smoke and have other positive health parameters pay less for life insurance.

A number of my patients, who work for larger companies, participate in programs that provide incentives for regular health evaluations and tests. Patients bring in a one-page form for the doctor to fill out, entering details of blood pressure, height and weight, cholesterol and blood sugar levels, urine values, etc. The doctor signs the form, sends it back to the company, and the worker receives either a cash rebate (like $300) or pays a lesser monthly amount as their share of insurance.

As individuals, we can begin this reform effort by taking the best care of ourselves, and also by working with our team of healthcare providers. As doctors, we can provide encouragement in offering a type of practice focused on motivation towards health rather than just disease treatment; also by offering ongoing education to support improved wellbeing. In other words, **get health care to support care for health.** These steps, along with some government regulations and cost controls, will make significant progress towards improved health for both individuals and society.

This NEW Medicine approach begins with addressing the shift in a common attitude that the system should take care of us no matter what, no matter how, we care for ourselves. We all can benefit by being self-responsible and by using healthcare providers and the system to evaluate and support our health.

The time to act is NOW to avert the potential healthcare challenges that loom before us. To delay further will most certainly assure that future generations will face a continuing decline in the resources necessary to achieve and sustain their health, because:

The Stakes are Too High

The Consequences of Inaction are Too Great

The Benefits of Real Change are Too Compelling

Clearly, we are at a crossroads in our search for optimal health and health care and its application for each of us as individuals and for our society as a whole. Our dilemma is that many of the discoveries and policies that have made us an advanced and affluent society contain elements that can prevent us from maximizing the health outcomes of our own lives and the lives of those we love and serve.

What is needed is a practical and sustainable approach to solve our healthcare crisis—one that is health-based, multi-disciplinary, and involves a core focus on preventive education, encouraging patients to become active participants in creating their own health rather than passive recipients. Education is so important to the changes required. We need to re-incorporate the traditional role of the doctor as a teacher and educator.

This is my calling, the culmination of my career so far, beginning with my training as a conventional Western doctor, followed by an intensive study of the systems of Natural and Eastern medicines. I feel it is time we returned to some of these more traditional sources of healing that may have been ignored during the last decades of scientific and technological advances. **We are drawing together the varied threads of healing throughout the ages and across cultures, to weave together a new form of health care that embraces the very best we have accomplished as a species to advance the health of our own bodies and minds, of those in need around the world, and of the Earth herself.**

CORE CONCEPTS
OF THE NEW MEDICINE APPROACH

• Increased personal responsibility for sustainable health

• A focus on prevention and regular health check-ups

• Education and support for building health-enhancing habits such as better overall dietary and other lifestyle choices, especially with childhood education to enhance lifelong health awareness

• Improved Doctor-Patient Partnerships in caring for individual health

• Shifting our policies, laws and corporate priorities from a disease-focused approach to a preventive and health-supportive model.

• Financial incentives by the government and/or the insurance companies for changing bad habits, such as nicotine use, lack of exercise, etc., by lowering premiums or financial rebates for those who make changes or demonstrate lifestyle choices that support disease prevention and improved health.

CHAPTER 1

WHAT IS NEW MEDICINE?

N.E.W. is an acronym for the integration of three healing modalities:

N – Natural   E – Eastern   W – Western

NEW MEDICINE OFFERS an integrated vision, empowering you to take more responsibility for your health. It presents an innovative synthesis of more traditional healing practices with the current "conventional" medical system. This integration, that is also offered at my clinic, combines a number of healing modalities and disciplines, including:

- Time-tested Natural and Eastern energy approaches to preventing illness and optimizing health

- Nutritional and Herbal medicines

- Cutting edge health psychology, wellness and lifestyle counseling

- The best of Western diagnostic technologies and pharmaceuticals when needed, as well as newer integrative testing.

NEW Medicine supports both practitioners and health consumers to learn about employing more effective health care toward better possible outcomes, with lower costs and long-lasting results. This approach encourages a fundamental relationship of preventive and integrative care between patient and doctor, and helps achieve improved health outcomes for various medical conditions, by helping each patient learn what's needed for their health and self-care strategy. This involves guiding people to discover what works for them to live most healthfully, choosing wisely, and employing natural remedies where possible. **Ideally, the goal is to do what works best in the most cost effective way and with the least toxicity.** This will benefit individuals and our society as a whole in controlling some of the rampant costs of providing health care.

This book explores and integrates many ancient healing practices; it is "NEW Medicine" because it brings time-tested healing traditions into today's healthcare practice, increasing the potential to be our best FUTURE Medicine. NEW Medicine can also be seen as good commonsense medicine, yet, it's more than that since what is presented here is balanced by scientific research. We already know what contributes to better health—follow a good diet and a healthy lifestyle that includes daily exercise, restful sleep, and other healthy habits, plus manage excess stress, and maintain a healthy attitude toward your life in caring for the only body that you have. NEW Medicine encompasses our relationship to self, loved ones, community and our planet.

"Ultimately, if we want to fix American medicine we will need skeptical and smart patients to dominate. They will need to ask the hard questions, because much of medicine is just plain old logic. So I am out there trying to persuade people to be those patients. And that often means telling them what the establishment doesn't want them to hear: that their answers are not the only answers, and their medicine is not the only medicine."[1]

—DR MEHMET OZ

One main premise about health is *"How we each look and feel is primarily a result of how we live—our lifestyle."* So our health care ideally focuses on evaluating and adapting our diet, exercise program, stress and sleep, relationships and work, and developing positive attitudes about our life and health. **This process is a primary principle for all practices of medicine and health care.**

Before proceeding let me ask you to do a brief check-in and assess your current approach to your health. Some good questions for self-review about your overall health and lifestyle include:

- Am I happy with my health and vitality?
- What can I do to optimize my health?
- Where do I need to make changes—diet, exercise, stress, etc?
- How can a healthier lifestyle support or improve my overall well-being?
- How familiar am I already with each of the NEW systems?
- Is my attention to my health based on prevention or crisis?
- What can I afford to be healthy?

NATURAL MEDICINE

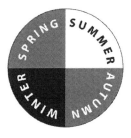

The quartered cross symbol represents Natural Medicine because the four seasons and the cycles of the year are the basis of the natural world and the healing it offers.

Natural Medicine has a long history throughout the world. Before modern medicine, Nature was all we had to rely upon to heal us. Today, this form of health care includes not only the use of appropriate medicines, but it also involves lifestyle, self-care, a nourishing diet, and ideally the guidance of a health practitioner for the use of naturally-based nutritional and herbal supplements.

Natural Medicine means reconnecting with Nature. This includes taking notice of the cycles of life, our local environment, and the changing seasons, as well as learning about the products of Nature and how to use them to rebalance and heal the body while doing no or little potential harm to the body or environment.

Since nourishment is an essential building block of good health, nutritional knowledge and its proper application are the keys to Natural Medicine. Ideally they are an essential part of each person's self care as well as a part of every primary care practice and training courses for our healthcare providers. My clinic has a knowledgeable nutritionist who specifically counsels and supports patients in regard to dietary changes pertaining to their health conditions. A comprehensive evaluation includes counseling about healthy food shopping and preparation of balanced meals for the individual and family. Ongoing support is essential to ensure that patients can make manageable changes in their eating programs and to help them remain healthfully motivated.

EASTERN MEDICINE

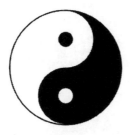

The Yin Yang symbol represents Eastern Medicine because it is an essential concept of this system, relating to the duality of life itself and to the inter-connectedness of all things.

Eastern Medicine is based on the ancient medical therapies from Asia. Terms such as Classical Chinese Medicine, Traditional Chinese Medicine, and Traditional Japanese Medicine refer to this style of medicine. Therapies include the various acupuncture techniques, manual body therapies, and herbal medicine practices as well as traditional energy exercise therapies, such as Qi Gong and Tai Chi.

Acupuncture is based on an ancient knowledge that recognizes a network of channels (meridians) coursing through the body and carrying vital energy called Qi ("chee"). This is understood as the life force that influences organ function, blood and fluid regulation, vitality, and the nervous system. All aspects of life—including stress, emotions, outdoor climates, as well as food, lifestyle and disease conditions—affect the vital force of Qi.

My first book, *Staying Healthy with the Seasons*, explains how the seasons and lifestyle affect health from the perspective of Eastern Medicine. It recommends seasonal acupuncture treatments as preventive medicine, as well as for pain and injury. Chronic conditions and imbalances may also respond well to acupuncture, helping to vitalize organ function that has become compromised. Eastern Medicine is more subtle in contrast to Western approaches. Also, it may take many treatments to achieve noticeable results as it builds on the body's preexisting conditions, helping to change them with no harm to the body. Over time, the body improves and becomes more resilient.

WESTERN MEDICINE

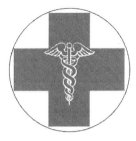

The Caduceus, two serpents entwined around a winged staff, is a common symbol of Western Medicine. The cross represents emergency care, which is a strength of this system, primarily using tests, drugs and surgery.

Western Medicine is our modern, technology-based system and is currently the predominant form of health care in the US and most Westernized countries. Acute care, trauma medicine, surgical interventions, and treating bacterial infections with antibiotics are the strengths of Western Medicine. I was initially trained in this system and use its basic principles to evaluate patients with physical exams, laboratory tests, as well as x-rays, ultrasounds, CAT scans and MRI's (when needed) to look into the body at the organs and tissues. There are also new types of testing for gut function, salivary hormones, food allergies, nutrient status, and measurement of the body composition, such as body fat, muscle mass, cellular hydration, and more. These can help physicians and patients to expand their medical repertoire by seeing in more detail how the body systems are functioning.

Drug prescriptions are a main part of Western medical practice. With a NEW Medicine approach, prescriptions are given when that is the most appropriate choice for what ails patients. As a "collaborative" or "cooperative" physician, I often write prescriptions when that's what the patient requests (after our review) as I believe that patients have the final say on how they treat their bodies, especially when they are well-informed. For example, a prescription medicine may be appropriate for depression that has not responded to lifestyle changes and natural therapies. Overall, my goal is to use less pharmaceuticals than the typical Western physician with a focus on creating long-term recovery and sustainable health with minimum toxicity and cost.

THE NEW MEDICINE SYSTEMS IN GREATER DEPTH

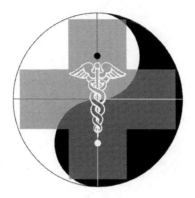

Now let's look more closely at the individual systems of healing—Natural, Eastern, and Western—that comprise NEW Medicine and see how they each work, and how to integrate them into one healing system.

- What are these three healing systems?
- How are they used and integrated?
- What are their strengths and weaknesses?

In most cities in America and in the Western world, you can find practitioners of conventional Western medicine as well as those who practice Natural or Eastern medicines in addition to local, ethnic traditional healers. In my view the wisest practice would use an integrated approach with some knowledge of all three systems and the appropriate application for every patient, allowing the simplest, safest and most effective treatments, which can then be adjusted over time as healing changes occur.

Currently there are also other healing practices that include homeopathy, chiropractic and other structural therapies, and electromagnetic (energetic) assessments and treatments. All of these modalities are potential components of a natural and complete medical system.

NATURAL MEDICINE

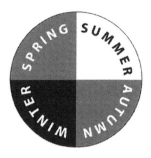

Natural or Naturopathic Medicine (NM) refers to traditional therapies that are derived from Nature, including a diet centered on healthy foods, naturally-derived supplemental nutrients and herbs, as well as body therapies such as massage and structural alignment (see more on structural therapies later in this chapter). People practicing natural medicine include: Naturopathic Doctors (NDs), nutritionists and dieticians, chiropractors, acupuncturists, herbalists and some MDs (Medical Doctors) and DOs (Doctors of Osteopathy). NDs are primarily focused and trained in this system, whereas other practitioners pick it up as an additional part of their training, or with special courses, many as CEUs (Continuing Educational Units).

Licensed Naturopaths receive a doctoral degree (ND) in these forms of therapy by completing a four-year program in clinical naturopathy. Those without a degree in natural medicine are usually trained through individual classes or certification programs. Nutritionists or nutritional counselors have various degrees of training on the effects of different diets and in how to eat healthfully along with the use nutritional supplements. They are not trained the same as dieticians, whose focus is more on medical diets for disease condition such as diabetes and cardiovascular problems. The thousands of nutritional supplements and herbal products found in the market-place today can be confusing to most lay people without the guidance of a knowledgeable practitioner of natural medicine, and how these apply to an individual's health needs.

How does this approach apply to us as individuals? It helps for each of us to know our body and to have an experienced natural medicine practitioner on our healthcare team, or can we learn online from a wide variety of sources.

WHAT IS A NATUROPATH?

In recent years, there has been an ongoing debate about the term Naturopathic Doctor (ND) between the 4-year clinical schools, which are more like conventional medical schools, and those without clinical programs, that also teach the principles and systems of traditional naturopathy. and may also offer an ND title after their students' names.

Most states acknowledge the ND practitioner and some do delineate between the different classes of qualification. This can be confusing to clients and needs to be sorted out in the coming years. My suggestion is to provide two different sets of titles: first NMD (Naturopathic Medical Doctor), for the clinical practitioner; and second, ND, or perhaps NME for Natural Medicine Educator.

In the meantime, as a consumer, it may be important to know which kind of ND you are working with.

Natural Medicine is based on the premise that the body has the innate ability to heal itself. As NM often uses nutrients and remedies that are specific and natural to the body, it has the potential to stimulate inherent, built-in mechanisms to repair and rebalance our body, mind, and heart. Natural Medicine is also a term that embraces *Physiological Medicine*, or what many physicians who incorporate Nature-based therapies into their practices call *Functional Medicine* or even *Integrative and Holistic Medicines*. This basically means maintaining or restoring healthy functions to the cells, tissues, organs and entire body.

FOUR TIMELESS PRINCIPLES OF NATURAL MEDICINE

• **"First, do no harm"** is a basic precept of Hippocrates, the father of modern medicine, and it is an essential part of Western medical doctors' graduation credo. This maxim certainly applies also to NM and EM, maybe even more so, since they both provide less dangerous treatments overall. In modern medicine this means using low risk procedures and healing substances, such as dietary supplements, herbal and/or homeopathic remedies, good water and hygiene, and hands-on treatments. Also, not doing harm means using the safest products possible, even drugs when lifestyle and natural therapies are not sufficient. **It also means reviewing the risks versus potential benefits before applying any treatment.**

• **Let Nature be the source of health** and healing by removing barriers that interfere with our own natural healing abilities and processes and by providing natural elements that we are designed to utilize.

• **Identify and treat the cause of illness** rather than use artificial medication to suppress symptoms that might lead to an accurate diagnosis, or may even be the body's attempt to generate healing, such as a fever with infection or the release of mucus during a cold.

• **Customize each treatment plan to fit the particular patient,** eliminating adverse effects that can occur with standardized protocols, and keep adjusting treatment as healing progresses.

Natural Medicine emphasizes education so that people learn to take care of themselves and recognize early signs of illness and prevent the development of chronic disease. In diagnosis, the whole person is taken into consideration rather than specific symptoms alone. Each patient is considered unique in physical, mental, emotional, social, sexual and spiritual aspects. Therefore there is no "one size fits all" approach. Protocols that work well for one patient may not be appropriate for others. Natural medicine recognizes the unique aspects of each individual's genetic background and environmental history and the influence these may have upon their susceptibility to disease as well as their individual innate healing abilities. Relationships also have an effect on our health, for better or worse.

Natural Medicine practitioners view the body as a whole organism, not merely a collection of organs and tissues. They also acknowledge that environmental factors, such as chemical exposures and electromagnetic stress, can have a negative impact on healthy body function. *Everything is connected*—the body with the earth and environment--and Natural Medicine seeks to maintain that optimal balance and connection. Our bodies and our health are reflective of our personal and local environments. Everything we are exposed to physically, emotionally and psychologically has an effect upon our health and our ability to maintain it.

Practitioners trained in both Natural and Western Medicines may assess a patient's health using targeted diagnostic tests such as basic biochemical blood and urine testing (similar to WM). Also, looking at nutritional status and hormone levels (through blood, urine or saliva tests) may help find imbalances and offer some guidelines for improving health, which is a bit different from conventional WM.

TREATING SYMPTOMS OR ADDRESSING CAUSES?

Typically, from the NM perspective, medical problems are not isolated to one part of the body or only due to a germ invasion, nor are symptoms just meant to be treated or suppressed. Most symptoms can be looked at as messages of deeper health imbalances. Addressing the underlying imbalances and correcting them is the focus of an integrated NM approach. In other words, Natural Medicine operates from the idea that the best kind of medicine identifies the actual cause, or causes of, a medical problem, then applies natural approaches whenever possible to ensure lasting results.

For example, instead of just treating high blood pressure with an anti-hypertensive medicine, an NM practitioner would look at the entire lifestyle as a potential contributor, address any underlying issue of inflammation, and recommend a low-salt, weight reduction diet if weight is an issue (note: some people with hypertension are not salt sensitive or overweight).[2] Herbal medicines like hawthorn berry or motherwort might be suggested, and minerals such as potassium and magnesium might also be recommended. Of course, a fitness program and stress management are essential for everyone, and especially people with "hyper tension," i.e. too much tension.

Prescribing thyroid, adrenal, or sex hormones (including estrogen, progesterone and testosterone) may also be part of a natural approach, especially when using what are termed "bio-identical hormones." These are the same biochemical compounds that our body makes (or did make before aging) as opposed to synthetic hormones, which are not bio-identical and often create more side effects. Further research is needed however to demonstrate that bio-identical hormones are better or safer.[3]

My upcoming book, *NEW Medicine Solutions*, discusses these topics in greater detail with chapters on Healthy Aging and Hormones.

NM practitioners may also seek to understand the energetic balance of the body, and many of them are also trained in acupuncture and other energy therapies and treatments many of which may not be covered with basic health, or disease, insurance.

HERBAL MEDICINE

Herbal Medicine is the most widespread Natural Therapy worldwide. Almost all cultures, from the earliest times to the present, sought and passed on knowledge of local plants and their effects on human health and disease. In many cultures the indigenous healers were often herbalists, and this is true today as well. Learning about the healing properties of local plants is widespread and there are many teachers and schools of herbal studies. There are also many useful online resources such as The National Library of Medicine,[4] and The American Botanical Council.[5]

In the US there are national standardized examinations to test for herbal medicine knowledge to ensure accurate and safe herbal prescribing by practitioners. These certifications in herbal medicine are offered through the American Naturopathic Medical Certification Board.[6]

Nutrients and herbs, most of which are part of the plant kingdom, have been studied and used for centuries for their healing properties. Others have only become available more recently. There is an extensive body of ancient folk medicine and current knowledge about the effects of various leaves, roots, berries or flowers to help cure the body's ills and generally to promote wellness. Examples might include various ginsengs for energy and stress management, or ginkgo leaf and ginger root to enhance circulation and brain function. Drinking brewed teas is an excellent way to use herbal therapies. A wide variety of herbs and herbal combinations are also available in capsules or tinctures (alcohol and alcohol-free extracts).

Besides the natural/herbal therapies, lifestyle, diet and energy approaches, NM practitioners have many other tools in their "medicine" bag. For example, detoxification programs, juice cleansing and fasting (animals frequently fast instinctively when they feel sick) can be quite helpful in addressing health problems. Other NM treatments can involve hands-on therapies to rebalance the body structurally, because healthy physical alignment allows the energy to flow correctly, which usually promotes better health. This idea of energy flow and function is also a basis of Eastern Medicine. With structural medicine, the alignment of the bones of the spine (neck and back) with no impingement on the nerves is important to health and an energetic, pain-free body. In Western Medicine the idea of energy circulation is not generally embraced and the concern is more with blood flow as important to health. Lymphatic flow is considered important by all systems as it supports immune function and healthy detoxification and protection from germs and other toxins. Exercise is key to helping the lymphatic flow, as well as blood flow, of course.

NATURAL MEDICINE: STRENGTHS AND WEAKNESSES

Time has proven the benefits of Natural Medicine as the medical application handed down by our ancestors. These local nature-based remedies have worked for healing or lessening a condition, which by definition, was our first form of healing (since all we had was nature) and is part of every indigenous healing system around the world. Thus, every culture has its local plants and healers. For all of its antiquity, NM and herbal therapies are being shown today to work well when incorporated into a full system of modern medical care. In fact, most of our modern pharmaceuticals have herbal origins, such as aspirin based on white willow bark and digitalis from the foxglove plant. NM is a key factor in optimizing our individual lifestyle and becoming more connected to Nature. It supports health and does not usually stress the body as much as harsh, stronger drugs. There are often complementary or added effects when using nutritional and herbal products that can work well together without as many adverse effects. Yet, this does not mean that some natural medicines are not without side effects or reactions, such as allergies or digestive upset. In addition, many natural products can interact with pharmaceutical agents being taken. More science must be done to study possible adverse reactions. One known example is the effect grapefruit juice has on the assimilation and utilization of many drugs, wherein it prolongs the time in the body for some drugs and shortens it for others. Thus, as with any medical care, herbs must be used with knowledge and experience, along with advice from a trained healthcare professional, and reviewed with follow-up feedback.

Plant-based medicines, however, are typically not as strong or concentrated as pharmaceutical drugs, and thus, are often slower acting and take longer to affect a result. Admittedly, this can be an issue when people are acutely ill or in pain. Then, they want more immediate relief, and that's often where Western medicines come in handy; as medications usually have stronger physiological effects (as well as more potential side effects). There are countless examples of this. Herbal drinks and teas that may be helpful, toning and cleansing could include peppermint, ginger, garlic, rosehips and others along with a little lemon or lime, cayenne and honey.

Herbs and nutrients may have stronger and more immediate results when used at higher, therapeutic doses. Taking several caps a day or as directed may be stronger than drinking an herbal tea, and may have greater and quicker benefits. This can also apply to use of Vitamin A and C for fending off viral issues, or herbal tinctures for a variety of ailments. Of course, learning proper amounts and the basics of nutritional medicine allows this system to work most effectively. It is also essential to stay attuned to your own body to see what works best for you.

The popularity of Natural Medicine during recent decades has led to the production of a huge array of natural products available in our local food stores and many other venues. With more comprehensive therapeutic programs, these products can be quite costly, especially when used on a regular basis over months or years. To make matters more complex, many large pharmaceutical companies are now producing special nutritional products, such as omega-3 fish oils and healthy bacteria (*probiotics*). So now the natural supplement companies have new competition, and the lines between pure "drug" companies and "natural supplement" companies is becoming increasingly blurred. Plus, none of them are really tested by the FDA (Federal Drug Administration) for their safety or accuracy in amount delivered, so we are left with the companies' own responsibility to make safe and effective products.

Another current downside of the NM approach is that many insurance programs do not cover natural medicines or its therapies, whereas they do support and pay for the more expensive pharmaceutical drugs. (Note: Health Savings Accounts (HSAs), more commonly cover natural remedies with pre-tax dollars if they are set up accordingly, which often means they must be prescribed by a practitioner.)

PRESCRIPTION POLITICS

The politics of coverage between WM and NM is still going on between the government, insurance companies, and drug companies, who are making mega-billions on their highly marketed and at times questionably beneficial drugs. In spite of the fact that nutritional and herbal supplement companies have grown over the years, they can hardly compete with the pharmaceutical companies with their active lobbyists and million-dollar marketing budgets to influence both doctors and consumers to buy their drugs.

NATURAL MEDICINE—REVIEW

The strength of NM is in keeping people healthy by educating them about lifestyle and wellness, and helping correcting basic body imbalances, such as inflammation, which often manifests as symptoms and eventually as illness. One current weakness in NM lies in the lack of potency, purity, and consistency (of quality and dosages) of the active ingredients in available remedies, which may not be strong enough to treat people when they wait until they are quite ill to seek treatment.

We can act proactively to reduce illness and improve outcomes of treatment. For example, when we treat a cold early on with fresh garlic or chicken soup, sweating and rest, increased amounts of vitamins A and C, and herbal remedies, we may knock it out before it takes hold and worsens. Still the typical insurance coverage often does not pay the cost of NM visits, treatments, or remedies, whereas it almost always covers more expensive crisis care, even when people have been irresponsible with their bodies and their health.

NATURAL MEDICINE

Strengths

- Relative Safety
- Compatible with Body Chemistry
- Supports Innate Healing Energies
- Works Gently
- Less Expensive (usually)
- Long History of Human Use

Weaknesses

- Often not strong enough for more intense illness or pain
- Unregulated—so effectiveness and purity are issues
- Not much supporting scientific evidence
- Takes more time to act
- Can be expensive for long term programs
- Not typically covered by insurance
- Possible allergic reactions or contra-indications with drugs

The artwork in the upcoming Eastern Medicine section is adapted from my book *Staying Healthy with the Seasons*, published by Celestial Arts/Tenspeed Press, Berkeley, CA. 1981/2003.

EASTERN MEDICINE

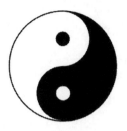

Eastern Medicine (EM) from Asia, especially China and Japan, is now an accepted form of treatment in the US. This ancient system of healing is many thousands of years old and is based upon a philosophy that views the body as an integrated energetic system that is synchronized with nature and its elements. Multiple channels called "meridians" carry vital energy that flows throughout the body. Along the body's skin surface, there are precise "points" that allow access to the energy system within the body. This bioelectrical energy is referred to as "Qi" (pronounced "Chee"), which is vital to the function of the whole body system. Any interruption to this network of channels affects the body's intricate healthy balance.

Imagine the meridians as a system of channels that crisscross the body similar to how multiple rivers flow in a landscape. There are 14 main meridians and their corresponding organ systems: Lung, Large Intestine, Stomach, Spleen, Heart, Small Intestine, Urinary Bladder, Kidney, Gallbladder, and Liver, along with the Pericardium, Three Heaters, Conception and Governing vessels (the latter four are not organs, yet affect energy systems). If any of these rivers,

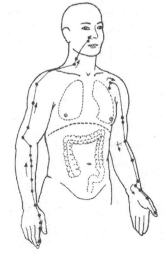

Large Intestine Meridian   Lung Meridian
Note: Meridians run on both sides of the body

or meridian channels run dry, or become dammed up over time, the consequences create adverse health events. Ideally every channel flows and functions smoothly without an interruption of the flow of Qi.

The practice of EM is also related to how the vital function of the body is in harmony with the natural elements and cycles that surround and influence us. This includes daily, monthly, seasonal and annual cycles. The internal climate of the body is influenced by the external climate and conditions as well as emotions, foods and stress. Typically, an EM practitioner reads the body's signs and evaluates symptoms through a variety of methods, such as "listening" or feeling the pulses at the wrist and assessing the person's smell and coloration of their tongue, eyes, cheeks and lips as well as palpating the abdomen and energy points. (There are also "alarm points" that can be tender when there is stress or congestion in certain organs or meridians.) After this assessment or diagnostic reading of the body, an acupuncture treatment and herbal formula is recommended.

HISTORY AND EDUCATION

Ancient texts written thousands of years ago outline the origins of Eastern Medicine. The fundamental doctrine called the "The Yellow Emperor's Inner Classic" is a historical account of health questions and answers that are presented as a dialogue believed to have taken place in the third millennium BC, between a revered Chinese emperor (Huang Qi - the Yellow Emperor) and his trusted health ministers. In this ancient text, the Yellow Emperor asks his doctor many questions about the pulses, how acupuncture helps diseases, and practical questions about the seasons, food, climate, emotions, diseases and how to live in harmony with nature. This "Inner Classic" actually consists

THE CHI CLOCK

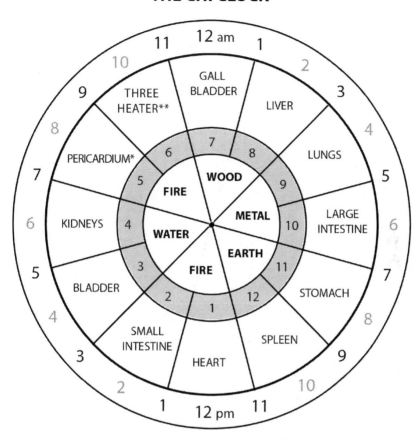

Each of the meridians is associated with an organ system and a time of day. Pericardium (also known as Circulation-Sex) and the Three Heater (or Triple Burners) meridians are part of the Fire element and work for body warmth, but are not associated with specific organs. This Chi clock does not include the Conception and Governing Vessels, which go up the front and down the back midlines of the body.

of two books, *Su Wen (Basic Questions)* and *Ling Shu (Divine or Spiritual Pivot)*, that answer many questions regarding the fundamental theory and treatment in classical Chinese medicine. This epic text could be compared to the *Hippocratic Corpus* in Greek medicine or the Sanskrit texts that are the foundation of Ayurveda.[7]

There are other revered ancient books describing classical Chinese medicine plus the benefits of herbal medicines and warming therapies like "moxibustion." These include *The Shan Han Lun (On Cold Damage)* and *Jin Gui Yao Lue (Essentials from the Golden Cabinet)* that were written later. These books were a departure from the more ancient shamanic practice of medicine before that time, and provided a cohesive format to the practical use of their medicine.

The evolution of this ancient classical medicine continued in China until the Cultural Revolution, occurring in 1966.[8] This devastating political upheaval resulted in the Chinese government changing the old ways to modernize their country; this meant revising and diminishing the practice of the more ancient style classical Chinese medicine. The new practice of medicine incorporates a more westernized, analytical approach and it was reclassified as Traditional Chinese Medicine (TCM).

These new ideas of medicine were incorporated into all of the Chinese medical schools and universities enforcing a more standardized format of Traditional Chinese Medicine. TCM was brought to the US after President Nixon visited China in 1972, since he was very impressed with the effects of TCM. Traveling with Nixon was *New York Times* reporter James Reston, who received acupuncture in China after undergoing an emergency appendectomy. Reston experienced quick post-operative pain relief and decided to write about acupuncture upon returning to the United States.[9] This visit led to the greater acceptance of TCM as a valid healing system and eventually to the opening of accredited acupuncture educational programs in US schools and abroad. Interestingly, Japan and Korea were not significantly affected by China's cultural revolution and have preserved more of the ancient, classical teachings that were modified with China's modernization.

I was often teased or criticized by my medical colleagues when I first began incorporating EM into my practice in the mid-1970s, along with nutrition and detox programs. Now, they are often included in many medical practices and there is a modified course that western-trained physicians can take to certify them to practice acupuncture. Some insurance plans cover acupuncture and it is accepted as an effective program for drug detoxification, pain reduction and stop-smoking plans. I look forward to further progress.

In the US, there are several nationally accredited Traditional Chinese Medicine programs. These are post-graduate programs and include at least 3,000 hours of instruction and clinical training. Following the successful completion of a program, a national certification exam is required before a license can be applied for. Each state has its own licensing requirements to practice and maintain that license. More recently, a standardized doctoral level of training has been approved, requiring at least 1,200 additional hours including intensive internships in a specialty of medicine. These internships are often done in China or Japan. EM has also become more popular among medical doctors who can enroll in a shorter 700-hour program in order to practice acupuncture. They are not required to take the national certification exam or abide by state licensure, but have an abbreviated exam within their program.

An outline of the basic concepts of EM, or TCM, follows and a more complete overview is offered in my first book, *Staying Healthy with the Seasons*, as well as many other excellent books such as Ted Kaptchuk's classic *The Web That Has No Weaver*[10] and Efrem Korngold and Harriet Beinfeld's *Between Heaven and Earth*.[11]

KEY CONCEPTS IN EASTERN MEDICINE

Eastern Medicine is a holistic system based on keeping the body's energies and organ systems in balance; it is essentially aimed at prevention. This concept stems from the tradition in rural China, where village healers and their apprentices, often called "barefoot doctors," provided healthcare to the local population. They traveled through the rural areas providing the only medical care that was available. They treated emergencies as well as provided preventive care for pregnant women and children. In the ancient emperors' kingdoms the acupuncturists were paid to keep the wealthier people and royal families well.

Two concepts that are unique and fundamental to Chinese, or Eastern, Medicine are Qi (usually translated as "vital energy") and the yin and yang duality (the harmony of all the opposite elements and forces that make up our existence). These two concepts form what we might call the "roots" of Chinese medicine. Springing from these roots are the basic principles and theories about the dynamics of Qi and yin and yang, which form the "stems" of Chinese medicine. And resting on these principles is the rest of TCM theory and application, such as the causes of patterns of disharmony, which form the "branches."[12]

WHAT IS QI?

Qi, or Chi, is thought by some to be much like an electrical force/current that powers all circulating functions. Qi represents the vital force that keeps all of the organ systems healthy. Although it is not visible, just like electricity, its effects can be palpable and measured by functional MRI scans, bioelectrical scanners, and by observable clinical results.

Some of the most ancient concepts that support Eastern Medicine (EM) and its philosophy are derived from the book, *I Ching*, also called the "Book of Changes." It is an ancient source of information or practical wisdom that records how to understand life based on the changing energetic elements of nature. Its concepts regarding the two most powerful influences on our existence are referred to as Yin (dark, cooling, calming energy) or Yang (light, positive, and the warming, invigorating energy). Yin has also been referred to as feminine, receptive, passive, and cold, while Yang is masculine, excessive, active and hot.

According to these concepts, everything in nature is based on the balance between these two influential Yin and Yang forces. Over the years, there have been numerous interpretations of their meaning in everyday life, which describe major influences on how the body works, relative to their strengths and weaknesses. For instance, when a person has excess in the body, it is considered a result of something that is not controlling the condition. In the case of excess mucus, the digestive system may be underactive or deficient. Of course, not all body conditions can be explained simply, but this concept of the balance of Yin and Yang permeates the philosophy of EM and how the body functions and responds to influences on its health.

In review, Eastern medicine looks at the circulation of life force and how to keep it in balance. Natural yin/yang polarities can be seen in the light/dark cycles of day and night, the heat and cold of summer and winter, and so on. These natural dualities are complementary opposites—without one the other would not exist—and they are essential to life and health. However, in our electrically-lit, fast-paced, plugged-in world, we often lose connection with these natural cycles. Eastern Medicine helps us to incorporate the understanding of these polar opposites and how to create a balance between them for the total health of our body and mind.

The Five Elements with their Seasons and Colors

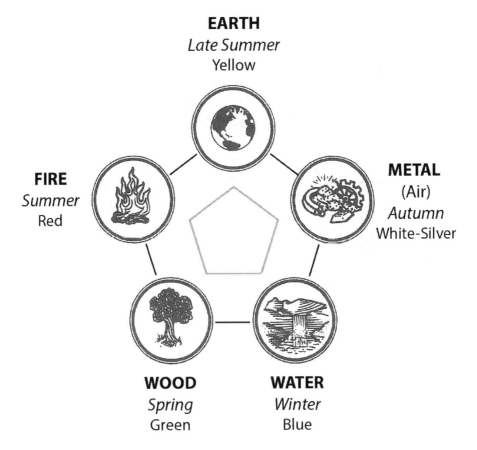

EARTH
Late Summer
Yellow

FIRE
Summer
Red

METAL
(Air)
Autumn
White-Silver

WOOD
Spring
Green

WATER
Winter
Blue

The seasons with their corresponding elements and qualities are at the core of Eastern Medicine's views of a holistic picture of the body, nature and the entire universe. These correlations are the key to how EM practitioners reach their diagnosis.

DIAGNOSIS IN EASTERN MEDICINE

When seeing a patient for the first time, the practitioner of EM uses a few essential tools to evaluate and determine a constitutional diagnosis and treatment plan. A health history is reviewed, and then the practitioner engages in a question and answer dialogue to learn of the patient's concerns and conditions. Observations are made regarding the person's speech, the power and tone of the voice, and the emotions associated with the words and conversation. How the patient looks and the nature of the "shen" or spirit helps to provide a deeper understanding of the person's condition.

Smell is another indicator used by an EM practitioner to help determine their body's constitution.

The "**shen**" or spirit is evaluated by the sense of comfort the person has within. It could include the color of the complexion, the clarity in the eyes, and the vitality of the energy or personality. This quality can be

Eastern Medicine diagnosis incorporates pulse taking, tongue observation, and body palpation.

When EM practitioners look at skin colors, they are assessing the elemental balance/imbalance related to the colors of the body elements and the corresponding organ systems.

There is also a sense of vitality or "shen," meaning spirit, which is expressed in the face, in the shade of the skin tone, its luminosity and the area surrounding the eyes. This is a significant part of the physical assessment and how the EM practitioner makes a diagnosis.

perceived only when there is enough time allowed for in depth exchange between the person and the doctor interviewing them, not usually found in a typical western medicine exchange.

PULSE DIAGNOSIS

An exam also includes a pulse analysis, in which the practitioner places their first three fingers along the edge of the patient's wrists just above their thumb, along the radial artery pulse. This wave of blood flow coming from the heart through the artery to the wrist has an ebb and flow motion that is detected by pressing along these three pulse positions. The quality of the pulse throbbing, the depth at which it is felt, and any irregularties in the rhythm of its beating are all detected with this exam.

Using pulse diagnosis (as an assessment tool) is the fine art of Eastern Medicine. It is based on a long tradition handed down from one master to another. Although it may seem subtle, the pulse palpation gives evidence not only of the variability of the pulse rate, but also to the strength and the quality of the blood and vital Qi. In contrast to Western medicine that feels the pulse to record its strength and beating rate.

The three pulse positions located on each wrist refer to different organ systems and are noted in their superficial and deep positions. There are many different relevant pulse findings, representing different conditions of organ systems that help in prescribing a treatment plan. For example, if the lungs and large intestine pulses are weak, the treatment may include a pattern of acupuncture points used to supplement these organ systems.

TONGUE DIAGNOSIS

There are distinct patterns that show up on the tongue that provide additional diagnostic information for the Eastern Medicine practitioner. The tongue's shape, size and color are noted as well as whether it has a coating. The coating may be thin or thick, ranging from white to dark and sticky or dry. It can change more quickly, however the size and thickness of the tongue is more consistent and helps determine a patients constitution, which is usually a lifelong pattern. There are often markings and cracks in the tongue body that reflects the body's imbalances or damage to vital fluids and organs.

BODY PALPATION (MANUAL EXAM)

TCM does not rely on body palpation as much as the Traditional Japanese acupuncture methods. In the Japanese system, the palpation of the abdomen, called the "Hara diagnosis," is a main source of diagnostic information. The abdomen is gently pressed to feel for hard and soft areas, or painful areas. This reveals where there may be deficiences and excesses in the organ systems. The extremities are also palpated, looking for sore spots and markings. The spine along the vertebrae is palpated as well and adds to a broader diagnostic picture of the patient. (Note: As a treatment Chi Ni San is a type of EM abdominal massage that can be helpful at reestablishing energy flow in the organs, helping with digestion and more.)

ACUPUNCTURE TREATMENT

The origins of acupuncture are documented more than 2000 years ago. The purpose of the acupuncture treatment is to tap into the connecting channels or meridians through selected acupuncture points to activate or balance the flow of Qi energy.

There are many styles and acupuncture techniques that are based on the unique teachings from China, and other Asian countries including Japan and Korea. Like most healthcare practitioners, each individual practices in his or her own distinctive way, using various techniques and technical skills. Each represents their profession in their own way and therefore some are more compatible with a given patient's needs or medical conditions than others.

ACUPUNCTURE IS OFTEN EFFECTIVE FOR:

Allergies	Fertility Issues
Anxiety	Headache
Arthritis & Joint pains	Hormonal Imbalances
Asthma	Irritable bowel Syndrome
Autoimmune diseases	Kidney Stones
Back & Body Pains	Menstrual irregularities
Constipation	Sinus disorders
Cough/Bronchitis	Sore Throat
Depression	Sleep disorders
Diarrhea	Tendonitis
Digestive disorders	Thyroid disorders
Dysmenorrhea (painful periods)	Urinary disorders
Ear and Hearing problems	*and many other conditions*
Fatigue	

The most common style of acupuncture uses thin 1 to 1.5 inch long stainless steel disposable needles. They are inserted through the skin into selected acupuncture points that are relevant to the meridian pathways of the specific organ systems being treated. They are usually inserted at a shallow depth of ¼ inch, or sometimes deeper to 1 ½ inches where there is more muscle mass. Japanese methods use needles that are relatively thinner and are typically inserted at a more shallow depth, and in some cases the needle is not inserted at all but merely held at the surface of the skin. Although even the thought of needles can elicit a pain response in some people, in reality acupuncture needle insertion is essentially painless. In fact, most treatments elicit deep relaxation that some people experience to be more restful than a full night's sleep. The treatment usually lasts from 30-60 minutes and it's not uncommon to fall asleep while lying on the table during treatment. Acupuncture may be effective with one treatment, yet some conditions may require a series of sessions to establish change and energy shifts in the body.

The National Center for Complementary and Alternative Medicine (NCCAM), now named the National Center for Complementary and Integrative Health (NCCIH), is an arm of the National Institute of Health (NIH). Since its start, it has funded thousands of studies and it still has a mandated budget measure for education. The center's research priorities include the study of complementary approaches, to manage pain and other symptoms that are not always well addressed by current conventional treatments.[13] These positive outcome studies have helped and now many insurance plans cover acupuncture.

The Center primarily funds research projects on what was once called "alternative medicine" including Eastern Medicine, acupuncture, herbal and nutritional strategies, mind-body health and more. NCCAM funded a meta-analysis of 29 randomized controlled studies on the effect of acupuncture on chronic pain in a total of more than 17,000 people, and they demonstrated the statistically significant benefit of acupuncture.[14]

There is now significant evidence that acupuncture used for some types of pain reduction increases endorphin levels, the molecules in our body that blunt our experience of pain.[15]

In general, acupuncture needles are either inserted into specific acupuncture points or into tender areas called "ashi" points—the tenderness is indicative of an area of congestion/stagnation of Blood or Qi. The needles placed in these points will relieve the tense or congested areas and allow for smoother flow of Qi through the channel. With experience and honed skills, these diagnostic techniques provide enough information to determine a diagnosis and a designated treatment plan.

In addition to using acupuncture, EM practitioners often apply heat to treat certain areas or conditions, either with an infrared lamp or a heated herb called mugwort or "moxa." The heated moxa can be applied on or around the acupuncture needle or directly on the meridian points. Sometimes a low frequency electrical current is used to stimulate the points or needles. Also once the needles are applied, the patient typically remains lying down for about 30 minutes before the needles are removed. Soft music may be played and the person relaxes deeply or may fall asleep.

Another way of treating the acupuncture points uses sound vibrations from medical tuning forks to stimulate the energy pathways. I developed and used this during my early work in the 1970s, and referred to it as *Sonopuncture*, or sound acupuncture, and in recent years, other ways of tuning the body with tuning forks have been researched and made popular by John Beaulieu[16] and others. The tuning fork sends a specific vibrational current into points affecting the Qi activity through the meridians, helping to clear energy blocks and supporting the energy flow. I know that tuning forks help people relax, and they often feel better and claim that their energy was flowing more freely. Perhaps our body is like an instrument being tuned? There are also light and color therapies being used on acupuncture points to stimulate energy movement.

EASTERN HERBAL MEDICINE

Similar to Natural Medicine, herbal medicine is also an integral and ancient part of EM. Although all the accredited acupuncture programs in the US include the study of both acupuncture and herbal medicine, in China doctors tend to specialize in one or the other. The Chinese herbal medicine is highly specialized and its formulary includes more than 350 commonly used herbs plus hundreds of others. Basic herbal formulas are recommended based on early descriptions of their uses for common constitutional conditions.

Additional herbs are added to every formula to treat each unique condition. The herbs are blended together according to their individual characteristics, indications, and precautions of use.

RESEARCH ON EASTERN HERBAL MEDICINE

There are credentialing agencies for practitioners of Chinese medicine and acupuncture, which also includes knowledge of Chinese herbs.[17] Remember that except in the case of direct complaints, the FDA does not closely regulate such products, so this causes some concern for consumers who don't know how to select and prescribe herbs for themselves.

Although there is some caution regarding the quality of Chinese herbs, in recent years the Chinese and US manufacturers have improved quality standards. There is also a growing trend of organic growing methods of Chinese herbs abroad and in the US that has increased their quality and availability.

In China numerous clinical trials have been conducted using herbal medicine and document favorable scientific outcomes in treating a variety of conditions. Herbs are prescribed, based on extensive research plus their time-honored, ancient traditional uses. There is also extensive ongoing research in the US funded by the NCCIH, (National Center for Complementary and Integrative Health) on the effectiveness of herbal remedies. Some herbs have been found to have highly effective bio-active ingredients considered for prescription use. One recent study showed that Chinese herbs plus acupuncture have been effective in diminishing unpleasant nausea due to cancer chemotherapy.[18]

Unfortunately even natural herbs can be dangerous. For example, Chinese herb ephedra (ma huang) is a very effective treatment for asthma; however, it was inked to serious health complications, including heart attack and stroke, and in 2004 the FDA banned the sale of ephedra-containing supplements.[19] These were most often used and abused for weight loss and performance (and energy) enhancement.

Prepared patented Chinese herbal formula medicines are available in many Chinese markets and herb stores where there may also be EM practitioners to make herbal formulations for customers. There are also several US-based companies manufacturing Chinese herbal formulas. These may be focused on improved digestion, prostate health, female hormone balancing, or specific EM diagnoses like wet or dry lungs, stagnant chi, or sluggish digestion.

Many traditional herbal formulas that were designed thousands of years ago by herbal scholars in Asia are still used today to treat the same medical conditions they were designed for. An ideal herbal formula prescription is based first on the constitution of the patient (reflecting the EM diagnosis) and then according to the condition and symptoms with which they are presenting. In essence, it takes into account the whole body, its weaknesses and strengths, while also addressing the current condition and illness.

Herbs are classified as food and in comparison are much weaker than a prescribed pharmaceutical drug. They are often recommended to take on a daily basis instead of as a short course of treatment. Many herbs can also be used in cooking. Common ones, like garlic and ginger, turmeric and oregano, can have a medicinal effect but also tonic herbs can be included in soups and broths to support the constitution. Integrating herbs into the diet as food and medicine supports the body's constitution and prevents the progression of illness. Creating the right combination of herbs to balance each patient's constitution is intrinsic to the art of an EM practitioner.

EASTERN MEDICINE REVIEW

Eastern Medicine is a highly developed system of natural medicine originating in Asia with its philosophy of cycles and seasons, energy reading of pulse vibrations, assessment of patterns of balance and imbalance through observation of various physical characteristics. The EM practitioner uses an elemental health analysis of the tongue's coloration and patterns, the eyes' health (vitality, brightness) and color hues in areas around the eyes, skin coloring and quality, the body's smell, and of course, the pulses. In some respects, when practiced by highly-trained experts, EM can offer additional levels of health assessment than those of the Western approach.

In general, EM seems to be a more subtle form of health care than Western medicines, which are usually faster acting and more directed at reducing symptoms. However, EM's effects are often cumulative, corrective and can be preventive over time, helping to reduce symptoms or the likelihood of developing a major illness. As with any kind of preventive care, similar to maintaining a car, the body performs best with regular checkups and maintenance. Initially, if there is a problem, treatments are recommended more often, like once to twice a week, while regular maintenance can be scheduled more periodically or according to the seasons. When signs of weakness or illness appear, early treatment ensures better results. Ultimately, if regular treatments are consistent, emergency breakdowns or serious illnesses are less likely to occur.

EASTERN MEDICINE:
STRENGTHS AND WEAKNESSES

Strengths-Advantages

- Safe and effective
- Gentle and relaxing
- Provides preventive care
- Relatively Inexpensive and may be covered by insurance
- Treatments can have a cumulative effect
- May result in less Western medications or reduces medication side effects
- Good for mental/psychological health and balancing mood disorders
- Can improve energy and sleep
- Often effective for pain

Weaknesses-Disadvantages

- Requires an experienced practitioner
- Not typically as effective for acute conditions other than pain
- Fear of Needles (can use acupressure, sound or heat instead)
- Not always covered by Insurance
- Requires multiple treatments

AN ACUPUNCTURIST'S PERSPECTIVE

Gigi Shames, LAc, is a popular acupuncturist at my clinic and graduate of Five Branches Institute in Santa Cruz, CA. Here she offers her comments related to her studies, practice and patient experience.

There are countless advantages and benefits of acupuncture, which I'm lucky enough to see every day. Yet, one of the concerns that some may view as a disadvantage regarding EM is more about how it is perceived in the Western/Allopathic medicine model. Its individualized treatment protocols do not fit a traditional Western research model of double-blind randomized, placebo-controlled clinical trials. In other words, when attempting to compare whether acupuncture relieves a migraine headache, for example, as effectively as Western medications, the allopathic MD may ask to see peer-reviewed articles on the efficacy of the acupuncture for the treatment of migraines. Because of its individualized treatment based on the patient's constitution and condition, one set of acupuncture points may not apply to the next patient with the same condition. In the allopathic research model, this allows a false perception of efficacy for those who base their medical decisions on the conventional research methods.

Taking the above example of migraine to illustrate further the individuality of EM therapies; there is not one "migraine treatment protocol" in Eastern Medicine, as the patient's constitution, pulse and tongue signs, and specific symptoms (pain location versus pain quality, what makes the pain worse or better etc.) determine the diagnosis and thus the treatment (to say nothing of customized herbal formulas). Therefore, when standardized treatment protocols for each migraine patient are used in allopathic studies on acupuncture's efficacy, the true nature of Chinese Medicine's strength is not fully being observed.

Yet, despite the inherent difficulty of fitting acupuncture into the parameters of conventional allopathic treatment models, EM performs well clinically with growing research studies funded by the National Institute of Health. It suggests that many medical doctors may not be reviewing these controlled studies about acupuncture and sometimes only recognize negative reports that may appear in popular media or random medical reports. EM continues to flourish among the health-conscious population as a wonderful integrative modality with a robust reputation and excellent results.

Eastern Medicine is a complex system with layers upon layers of depth beyond the seeming simplicity of some of its natural concepts. To become an expert practitioner in EM requires many years of study and practice. EM may also require several, even many, treatments to help correct some acute and chronic conditions, and this can be costly and time consuming. No system works all of the time, and often it takes a little learning curve for the patient/client/consumer to embrace the fine art of EM and realize its overall benefits.

WESTERN MEDICINE

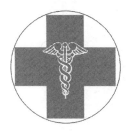

Western Medicine (WM) is the medical model that most of us are familiar with in the US. In theory, treatment is based on empirical science incorporating evidence-based research. The focus is on diagnosis and then choosing the best pharmaceuticals or surgery for disease management. However, even with research, individual responses vary such that the practice of medicine is more of an art that bases its practice on science. As already mentioned, WM has both great benefits and challenges. Before the modern era of Western Medicine, "Natural Medicine" was all we had. Staying healthy was an essential component of our daily lives. To be sure, early methods of health care had limitations, including medical decisions with diagnosis and treatment depending on superstitions, experience, and knowledge at the time. Very few effective treatments were available to battle serious infections and plagues, surgical tools and techniques were primitive, and technical ability to diagnose conditions was limited. Also, a century ago average life expectancy was about 50 years: infectious diseases were the primary cause of illness and death. Retirement wasn't even a fantasy then, nor was the idea of "seniors".

In past centuries and in non-Western cultures, the "doctor" had a very different role than now in the West, often serving as a combination of Healer, Teacher, Guide, and Counselor. Today, WM is BIG business, and "specialization" is the name of the game. Illness and chronic conditions often force doctors and patients into specific, isolating relationships, often with each particular symptom or body part taken care of by a different doctor.

How did we go from the physician embracing all the roles of healer and life guide to every symptom or condition requiring a different doctor? Certainly the explosion of knowledge and research about human biology has driven much of this specialization. Yet, in many respects this situation has also arisen from the business of medicine with its focus on technology, and so much information requiring medical specialization for adequate informed care, with insurance companies often dictating choices.

DOCTORS ARE OFTEN STRESSED AND UNHAPPY TOO!

Our modern Western Medical system also impacts the health of our physicians and other healthcare practitioners. Clearly, doctors today can become over-worked, depressed and frustrated with the stressful demands of medical practice and paperwork. Many doctors surveyed expressed that they were suffering from burnout and considering leaving medical practice in a few years.[20] In hospitals the situation can be even worse. Due to the numerous clinical errors from sleep-deprived medical interns and residents, new rules were established to prevent the traditional 30-hour overnight shifts and working 16 hours straight.[21] And there's a lot more paperwork or computer work to be in compliance with government and insurance rules and regulations.

Dealing with crisis after crisis and with challenging patients who often don't get better yet need consistent managing, is depleting both personally and financially. Ironically, this growing crisis is often due to the very fact that the Western Medical approach does not foster true healing. Real healing is the actual undoing of the problem in which causes are addressed and corrected; of course, causes are not always identifiable.

Western Medicine is also called "Allopathic," which means treating diseases and suffering by remedies that produce effects opposite to the symptoms, such as a pill to lower blood pressure or cholesterol, or a drug to slow the intestinal tract to stop diarrhea. It also includes counteracting suffering ("pathy/pathos"), such as reducing pain from inflammation or injury.

The Western system of medicine excels at eradicating a symptom or problem primarily with drugs and surgery—as when treating an infection with antibiotics and abnormal cancer cells with

> **Allopathy** is defined as "treatment of disease by remedies that produce effects opposite to the symptoms," from the Greek allos "other" + -patheia "effect." This term was applied to contrast with **homeopathy**, where like treats like.

chemotherapy, or removing or replacing a damaged body part. This approach primarily eliminates symptoms, which I refer to as the "attack and conquer" philosophy of Western medicine. Often the medications used are strong enough to achieve results, but can also create serious side effects.

Of course, WM isn't always just drugs and surgery. A more Integrated and Preventive Medicine component can be incorporated, which is how many doctors have advanced their practices in recent years. This includes education as an important part of practice, as well as supporting people in deciding the best treatments based upon their beliefs and desires, rather than doing things based solely on the doctor's decision or "science." What most Western-based doctors are practicing, I call *Conventional Medicine* (doing what's aligned with current convention). When other assessment and treatment modalities, such as nutrition and acupuncture, are incorporated, I use the term *Traditional Medicine* because it is based on long-standing traditions. The idea of **Integrative Medicine** comes from merging both conventional and traditional practices.

WESTERN MEDICINE—TESTS AND TOOLS

Current WM focuses on technological assessment of the body and its problems, employing physical exams, blood chemistry testing, various scans like x-rays or MRI's and then treating with pharmaceutical medicines or surgery. The following chart lists some tests that are routinely performed in WM, and the kind of information they provide. It incorporates standard medical testing as well as functional, integrative testing. In recent years, many new and innovative tests have become available to assist healthcare professionals in seeing if the body is functioning properly, such as looking at nutrient levels, and more subtle assessments of the body's imbalance and homeostasis.

Blood Tests: Complete Blood Count (**CBC**) provides information on the quantity and distribution of blood cells supplying clinical clues on the presence of infection, anemia, bleeding problems, or allergies; **Comprehensive Medical Panel** (**CMP**) measures such things as liver and kidney function, protein levels, calcium and electrolytes (sodium, potassium, etc.) and hormones such as estrogen or testosterone. Many hundreds of different tests are available to assess body function and chemistry.

Urine Tests: Looks at pH (acidity) and the kidney's ability to function, whether abnormal levels of protein, sugar, blood cells or microbes are present. The presence of blood cells or microbes could indicate an infection in the bladder and kidneys. Newer tests can look at urinary hormones, neurotransmitters, or heavy metals, chemical toxins and organic acids.

X-Rays and Body Scans—Ultrasounds, MRIs and CAT scans: Traditional x-rays can look at any part of body mainly seeing the bones. CAT (or CT-Scans) and MRIs can also examine the health of soft tissues like in the brain or the cartilage and tissues of the knees. These are newer, more complete (3D) views and are more costly as well as more radiation for the CTs, which can look for tumors and other tissue abnormalities. MRIs can show more soft tissue problems such as ligament or tendon tears, and can also pick up cysts, tumors and inflamed joints (as with arthritis). Heart Scans can be used to detect calcium plaque in the coronary arteries, and this is helpful for evaluating cardiovascular risk. Whole body scans are also used to screen the body for tumors and other problems.

Saliva Tests: These are newer and now more commonly used tests, which save blood and in some situations may give a more accurate picture. Saliva can reflect the tissue levels of hormones. The measurements for adrenal cortisol levels (four samples through the day) from salivary testing ordered with the physician are generally accurate, although some home testing, or tests on the internet, may not be as reliable.[22] Saliva may represent the actual levels of what's active in the tissues rather than what's attached to protein just passing from place to place and not actively functioning. This type of testing needs to be studied further.

Stool Tests (Digestive Analyses): These can be simple screens for the presence of blood, looking for tissue damage or colon cancer, as well as microscopic testing or culturing for bacteria, yeast or parasites. We can also examine the ability to properly digest foods and secrete proper levels of digestive enzymes and hydrochloric acid, as well as the microbial analyses. Since gut health and the "microbiome" (the microbial makeup in the bowels) is so important for overall health, these stool tests have become an important assessment in NEW Medicine.

Scopes, Endoscopy and Colonoscopy: With new fiber-optic flexible tubes, doctors can visualize the upper and lower intestinal tracts and see the mucous membranes to look for inflammation and ulcers, injury, polyps and other tumors in the gastrointestinal tract (and bladder, called Cystoscopy) as well as do biopsies or removals of polyps. All of these tests help us to make a plan to deal with earlier signs of disease and create more effective programs to remedy them.

Genetic Testing: This is relatively new testing and soon perhaps real Preventive Medicine to help look at our biologic risk factors and then address ways to reduce our risk and incidence (at least delay) the onset of these potential medical conditions. This is still mostly a research tool.

Note: Of course, tests can be invaluable in helping doctors and patients assess what's going on, yet too much focus on testing can lead to increased costs, misdiagnosis or over-diagnosis—finding things of no consequence like a kidney cyst that can lead to more unneeded testing, treatment and expense. Also, testing itself can cause some ill effects from blood draws, x-rays, or CAT scans that require injections of various substances like gallinium, thallium (more toxic), and technetium.

WESTERN MEDICINE AND PREVENTION

The drug companies and many Western physicians would have us doubt that options other than drugs and surgery actually do work. Let's face it: prevention isn't the most "profitable" for most practitioners. Prevention end points are hard to measure except across lifetimes. **NEW Medicine is a call to action to transform this paradigm by making integrative and preventive care an imperative.** Only we—as individual health consumers and doctors—can make this happen.

Several recent workplace wellness studies, such as for the Safeway employee programs, have shown that a dollar invested in prevention reduces future healthcare costs by several dollars or more. Of course, much of the initial data come from smoking cessation and weight loss programs to prevent tobacco or weight-related illnesses, which are measurable objective outcomes. Yet, numerous corporate employee benefits programs showed lower health care costs after the employees participated in a health behavior change program. And of course, they lowered their risks for subsequent illnesses. In other words, eliminating an objective negative behavior can lead to a positive health improvement that benefits each person and society as a whole.

Preventive Medicine clearly makes sense—the better our health as individuals and as a society, the better quality of life we have, the lower our healthcare costs, and hopefully, the lower our insurance premiums and the higher our productivity. **In concert with Natural and Oriental approaches, Western Medicine also has the capability to deliver Preventive Medicine to us all.**

What WM currently considers preventive care is primarily immunizations and screenings for illness risk factors with a focus on early diagnosis. Our current preventive model depends on measurable net benefits (which, ideally is the measure of any treatment, be it NM, EM, or WM), the level of certainty of the outcome and expected outcome due to a specific preventive measure. The Guide to Clinical Preventive Services are recommendations by the US Preventive Services Task Force—the people who research what works and what doesn't.[23] Here are current preventive WM approaches according to the guide:

- **Lifestyle Review**—regular screening for health behaviors (e.g. diet and exercise)

- **Obesity and weight guidance** with body composition (fat and muscle percents)

- **Smoking cessation programs** (plus other nicotine habits)

- **Cancer screening,** which involves mammograms, chest x-rays for smokers, colonoscopies, PSA tests for prostate, etc.

- **Heart disease risks** with lipid level measurements

- **Vitamin D** measurements and other nutrient levels for deficiencies

- **Vaccinations** and regular Flu shots

Nutritional supplementation recommendations may be suggested to prevent heart disease and cancer, as well as for healthy pregnancies and babies. It's all about screening. However, counseling for diet and behaviors are now on the guideline list with a focus on obesity screening.

All of this LOOKS good, but it turns out most clinicians often do NOT talk to their patients about weight or lifestyle issues; they don't have the time, plus they have not been taught much about how to do this. This is a fee for service issue *(charges based on specific face-to-face time with patients or for tests or procedures);* we need to have educators talk about healthy choices. Yet, times are challenging with our TVs and computers being used for health education, as well as phones, pads and Apps.

WESTERN MEDICINE: STRENGTHS AND WEAKNESSES

Without relying daily on advanced tests and treatments made available in current Western health care, including pharmaceuticals when needed, I could not offer the level of success and quality of health care that I now provide. When people are acutely ill or injured, or for those patients with advanced health problems, we could not relieve their pain and suffering without drugs and/or surgical procedures, nor could we determine what is wrong without appropriate testing. Thus, I am a wholehearted proponent of WM's strengths, many of which—when used judiciously in concert with Natural and Oriental approaches—can support our health and healthcare system as a whole.

Yet, as with Natural and Eastern Medicines, WM also has its shortcomings. It often treats problems too aggressively because a strong medicine might be all that the doctor has to offer to eliminate symptoms. When I began practicing medicine in the early 1970s, the medicines that were available often didn't quite fit the treatment needed or more commonly, the diagnosis was not always clear enough to indicate that the given drug was the right choice. This was partly why I began seeking out other systems that offered simpler, more natural and potentially helpful treatments. It seems that guiding people to optimize their weight and diet while learning how to manage life's stresses was needed to help correct the underlying problems that gave rise to specific symptoms or conditions. This awareness has led many physicians to study other systems and develop the integrated practice models we are now beginning to utilize. The NEW Medicine approach is a reflection of what we consider works best for many chronic problems and acute health issues. This approach allows us to address the underlying causes more readily and, collaboratively with the patient, develop a cost-effective implementable plan for optimal healing and health that also offers little risk of harm. For example, even though many drugs can lower high blood pressure, we cannot really correct and heal the underlying issue without changing the diet, or dealing with excess weight and stress management. When a person's lifestyle is simultaneously corrected while taking the appropriate medication, this may prevent further problems and expense.

Similarly, while surgery can be lifesaving, it can also be risky and life threatening, not to mention being exorbitantly expensive. This is one reason, unless it is for acute medical and/or surgical cases, we need to explore natural measures first and save surgery as a last resort. Many patients share this view.

WESTERN MEDICINE

Strengths

- Medicines are strong and effective
- Antibiotics for microbial infections when used correctly
- Surgery when used correctly
- Technology to assess the body
- Advances in technology
- Immunizations to prevent life-threatening infectious diseases

Weaknesses

- Medicines are strong and can cause other problems
- Drug interactions are not always known.
- Antibiotics when misused (e.g. for viral infections) which may compromise our immune system and gut microbiome and cause antibiotic resistance
- Surgery when not necessary
- Overuse of technology
- Medical/technical advances when they replace commonsense
- Immunizations and their adverse effects
- Does not solve/address root problems/causes
- Is mainly profit-driven and not "health" driven
- Over-specialization, few doctors left who treat the whole family or whole person
- Frequently critical of other forms of medicine, therefore diminishing adequate conversation/communication with patients

Another way to look at our dominant system is to consider a list of what Western Medicine is good for and what it is not. Dr. Andrew Weil summarized this in his engaging breakthrough book, *Spontaneous Healing*.[24] I paraphrase and integrate with added specifics:

Western Medicine is Good for (Advantages)

- Treating Bacterial Diseases
- Trauma Repair, i.e. Fractures
- Repairing damaged joints, knees/hips
- Diagnosing/Treating Medical Emergencies
- Treating Fungal and Parasitic Infections
- Diagnosing complex medical conditions
- Diagnosing/Treating hormonal deficiencies
- Cosmetic/Reconstructive Surgery

Not as Good for (Disadvantages)

- Treating Viral Diseases
- Correcting Chronic Degenerative Diseases
- Curing or Preventing Allergies & Autoimmune Diseases
- Treating Mood & Fatigue Issues
- Treating Mental Disorders Effectively
- Curing many forms of Cancer
- Using Natural Hormone Support
- Handling Stress and Psychosomatic Issues

OTHER INTEGRATIVE AND ENERGETIC THERAPIES

There are many other healing modalities and therapies that are a part of an integrated NEW Medicine approach, and in fact, many of these natural medicine systems have been used for decades, if not centuries. These disciplines span the physical, mental, psychological, emotional, spiritual and energetic aspects of individual health, and contribute to a truly multidisciplinary model of health care. These other systems of assessment and treatment include:

- **Structural Therapies**—Osteopathy, Chiropractic, Physical Therapy and Massage
- **Homeopathy**—Natural Therapies in Micro-Dilutions
- **Energy Medicine**—Electro-diagnosis and Treatment, Sound and Light Therapy
- **Mind/Body Healing**—Psychotherapy and Guided Imagery, Counseling and Stress Management, and Spiritual Healing

STRUCTURAL AND MASSAGE THERAPIES

Structural or "body" therapies are provided by many practitioners who are trained and experienced in using their hands (or other physical devices) for healing—in correcting, manipulating, and maintaining the structural integrity of the body. Keeping the body's spine, bones and tissues aligned helps the energy and nervous system to flow well for optimal health. Stresses, misalignment of the body, and injuries alter this integrity and can affect how well the nerves are enervating the tissues, influencing whether there is pain or good function in the area.

There are two primary licensed structural medicine practitioners: Chiropractors with a DC (Doctor of Chiropractic degree) and

Osteopaths, DO (a medical doctor with additional training in musculoskeletal treatment). Physical therapists (PTs) support many doctors and structural medical needs, and massage therapists (with a licensed CMT) are very popular form of structural therapy and most everyone loves a good massage. In Germany and Italy, going to a spa for massage and other body therapies is covered under their healthcare systems. Wouldn't that be nice here? Although it varies based on the practitioner's training and experience, massage generally focuses on releasing muscle and emotional tensions and relaxing the body/mind. Remember, everything is connected, and thus when the bones, muscles and other tissues are working well together, we can experience more vibrant health with less pain and with improved circulation.

Insurance coverage for the many different types of structural therapy varies a great deal according to individual policies. Coverage might depend on a physician's referral, the licensure of the practitioner, or the cause of the injury needing treatment, such as a car accident. Generally, Osteopathic Medical Doctors, Physical Therapists, and some Chiropractors are covered best by insurance companies. Some massage therapies are supported by a "flexible spending account" or "Health Savings Account" (HSA).

HOMEOPATHY

Homeopathy is its own system of health care that can be utilized with other systems as part of an integrated practice model, although some homeopaths prefer that it be used by itself without other therapies. From an American scientific perspective, it is not well understood or trusted, yet it does have many adherents who experience benefits and claim its good results, especially in European countries. It is taught in some European medical schools and is especially popular in the UK, where it has been covered by universal health care since 1948.

However, it is now falling out of favor and is not available everywhere. The National Health Service offers this treatment option primarily in its four homeopathic hospitals.[25] It is also said to be the form of alternative care most favored by European doctors.[26] The Queen of England and her family are said to use this form of medical therapy. It appears to work well when utilized according to its doctrines. Yet as stated, this is not well documented in scientific studies although it is very well documented by homeopaths themselves dating back to its foundation in the late 1800's. Some treatments work immediately with one dosage of a remedy, while others take time and require repeated dosages.

Homeopathy can used to treat most medical issues. We are also aware that according to the WM evidence-based approach, homeopathy is usually considered a placebo. Here's a deeper discussion to give you some of the primary aspects of this healing system.

Homeopathy is a relatively young system discovered and developed by Samuel Hahnemann in 1796. "Classical" Homeopathy, which follows a book of symptoms and remedies, known as the *Materia Medica*, is the most popular philosophical approach. Classical treatment is based on Hahnemann's original findings and testing of remedies, wherein he measured the effects and symptoms that each remedy caused in the body/mind when given to a healthy person. Then, he postulated that that these remedies would correct those same symptoms in ill people.

As the study of Homeopathy evolves, there are many who practice some variation mixing Classical with "modern" ideas and expanding the substances that can be used for treatment. Homeopathy may be used to help with acute illnesses and/or in a constitutional manner to help with deeper core healing for repetitive illnesses or diseases. As with Eastern Medicine, the success may be based on learning the constitutional and health state of the patient.

The idea of *"like treats like"* (thus the term *homeo*) is the basis for homeopathy (opposite of allopathic model, which tends to suppress symptoms by "opposite" treatment). For example, if you get a bee sting, you are treated with minute dilutions of bee venom. Dilutions may be so extreme that not even one molecule of the original substance is likely present. Homeopathic remedies, at low dilutions are sold as over-the-counter products, so they are accessible to everyone. The higher dilutions are thought to be more powerful and must be prescribed by a homeopath. A layperson might be able to figure out a remedy that would help in an acute illness or symptom, but since homeopathy is such a complex system, I recommend consulting with a trained homeopath to get the best results. Again, it is not a single symptom that is being treated, but often a constellation of symptoms. Plus, there is a constitutional remedy that works to strengthen the body, mind and spirit of an individual. Determining the constitutional remedy is a complicated process requiring time and expertise.

Within Homeopathy it is believed that the more diluted a substance/remedy is, the stronger its effects. The process of diluting homeopathic substances in a stream of water (and/or alcohol) to continually lessen the active ingredients is called *Trituration*. Stronger dilutions have actually no active ingredient, but only the energetic pattern (vibration) of the original substance.

Each dilution is followed by shaking the liquid preparation, called *succussion*, which is said to increase or activate the potency of the remedy. Homeopaths call this entire process *potentization*, These dilutions are then formulated into alcohol or lactose (milk sugar) tablets that easily dissolve.

DILUTIONS

Homeopathic treatment uses micro-dilutions of natural substances; the homeopathic drug potency is indicated on the label and is shown by a number followed by the letter X or C. The letter X indicates a substance base is diluted at a ratio of 1:9 (1 part active to 9 parts inactive— USP dilution alcohol). The ratio for a C potency is 1:99 (1 part active to 99 parts inactive alcohol). The number preceding the X or C signifies the number of times the base substance was diluted and succussed (agitated vigorously). The more a substance is diluted, the more potent it is. For instance, 200C is more potent than 30C. Although this is a bit counterintuitive, it is the basis of homeopathic treatment.

How can a little sugar (lactose powder) pill that contains no molecules of a supposedly active substance have any healing effect? Although many people, scientists included, have a hard time believing that such a substance could affect bodily or emotional changes, there are millions of people who claim great benefit from using homeopathy. From my perspective it is really a type of "resonance" or "vibrational" medicine for the body—shifting the imbalanced energies into a new state of harmony.

Many health food stores now carry low dilutions of homeopathic remedies used for insomnia, stress, and even to help prevent and fend off early flu (a popular product called *Oscillococcinum*). In the US homeopathy is often chosen for self-care by the educated individual willing to explore healing approaches other than allopathic treatment.

When doing a thorough diagnostic assessment, the homeopath considers the whole person (physical, mental, emotional, spiritual and energetic), and how that individual is uniquely presenting or expressing symptoms and imbalance. When a remedy is chosen that best matches the uniqueness of the person, then the remedy may be seen as reinforcing the healing process. The body is always seeking better balance. The strength of homeopathy is that it works with the body's own energy rather than against it. It also has minimal downside and side effects, yet some people may experience what homeopaths call an "aggravation," which is part of the healing process and suggests that a remedy is working. Homeopathy then may be especially useful for the sensitive patient, someone who can't tolerate stronger chemical medicines.

ENERGY MEDICINE: ELECTRO-DIAGNOSIS AND TREATMENT

Energy medicine is a broad term describing systems and methods of evaluating and sometimes treating the body in its many dimensions. Some are sophisticated, modern devices and instruments that measure electromagnetic points within and around the body, and test for responses. Some use acupuncture points to test the body. Examples of these instruments are the Electro-Interstitial Scanner (EIS) and EAV (Electro-Acupuncture according to Vohl, a German scientist).

Another example is Applied Kinesiology, a testing system that uses the person's own muscle strength to assess positive or negative body responses to questions about disease states and the benefit of potential remedies. Muscle testing has been used to look at potential allergic reactions, or to assess the best remedies for treatment, yet little research proves its objective value or benefit. Chiropractors seem to be the most common users of applied kinesiology and they use their adjustments and other treatments to do the rebalancing.

Many aspects of energy medicine assess what is out of balance to provide specific diagnoses about what's wrong in the body, from deeper infections, to immunization reactive patterns, to organ strengths and weaknesses. Assessing the energetic patterns of the body makes sense for the future of medicine, and this system aligns with EM, in that the energy flows are important to health and also that problems are seen to begin at the energetic levels before they become physical. Thus, assessing and correcting these patterns and balancing the energies in the body are more subtle ways to maintain health. This may be needed on an ongoing basis for maintenance or support of an existing injury or condition.

Although research doesn't offer much support for applied kinesiology testing and its results, it seems to be based more on the aligned beliefs of the practitioner and patient. Of course, belief plays a big part in our response to any treatment. In most studies the placebo effect is at least 30% and can be more than 50%. Western medicine and science, of course, look skeptically at energy testing as non-scientific.

SOUND, LIGHT AND AROMA THERAPIES

Sound, light, and color are pure energies/vibrations and they can influence and move body energies. The better we *activate* our body energies, the clearer and more vital we will feel. That's what acupuncture does—helps us move our electromagnetic energy. Sound and color therapy can also help in this. I have been involved with sound therapy for 40 years, having developed *Sonopuncture*, the use of medical tuning forks applied to the acupuncture system. This is based on an understanding of elemental imbalance and what specific points to use for improving balance, a treatment called *Sound Tune-ups*. People typically experience the vibration moving through the body and even along specific meridian channels. They can also feel an overall calming, peaceful feeling. Sound is a pure energy and can help heal. This also means using music and sweet, harmonious sounds to help soothe us.

"We become one with the cosmic symphony, as we are attuned and aligned in a rhythm renewal" —ARGISLE

Light therapy is also important and helps balance our cycles of light and dark, summer and winter. We are all affected by where we live on the planet and the kind of light/dark cycles and seasons that surround us. Many people use light boxes for depression and SAD (Seasonal Affect Disorder), and it can be helpful for resetting our body clock, brain chemicals, and neurotransmitters. I offer more about this topic in the Chapter on Energy and Mood Disorders in my upcoming book, *NEW Medicine Solutions.*

Aromatherapy is an increasingly popular treatment approach. We are all affected by any surrounding smells and aromas—from foods to herbs to oils and chemicals. Some influence us positively while others adversely. Clearly, they have some physiological affects and may benefit our health when applied appropriately.

MIND-BODY HEALING

Mind-body healing looks at the role that thoughts, beliefs, attitudes, and perception of stress play in our health challenges. Various approaches are used to become more aware of the mind's capacity to undermine our wellbeing or to achieve balance. This includes psychotherapy, hypnotherapy, guided Imagery, counseling, meditation, yoga and qi gong. A licensed psychotherapist may actually utilize all of these strategies to guide a person to achieve balance of mind and body.

One study of 845 cardiac rehab patients before and after a 13-week program in the Relaxation Response (a very simple meditation practice) showed that they had less depression, anxiety and hostility as well as enhanced spiritual wellbeing.[27]

Both emotional and mental levels of health are aligned with our physical wellbeing. Self-abuse, based on lifestyle actions/habits, is a common factor that can compromise health. Life's traumas and parental behaviors can lead us to believe that we are not worthy of love, which may cause us to treat our body disrespectfully, rather than with the love we deserve. A shift towards a better balance is so important to begin the step toward healing, as our personal attitude primarily represents how we choose to care for the only body we have.

Many behaviors, such as the overindulgence of common substances like caffeine, alcohol and sugar (and other potentially addictive substances or activities like TV, abusive relationships, etc.) are commonly accepted, as is the focus on work and lack of exercise and a general approach that places our health at a lower priority than many other endeavors in life. When we don't care for, or about our health, it and we, eventually suffer and deteriorate. When we consistently stimulate and sedate ourselves and have sleep or energy issues, we begin to rely regularly on artificial substances for help, and this leads to abuse and even addiction. One key issue here is that we aren't often aware of the detrimental changes until problems begin years later. We believe we're okay, but we're really not. In addition, lack of time or financial resources may keep us trapped in our stressful situations.

In regard to psycho-emotional health and NEW Medicine, it is important to remember that physical health is only part of our complex human equation. For people who have suffered physical trauma, emotional and/or sexual abuses, providing emotional and psychological support are essential first levels of care. It is a disservice not to explore other possible helpful therapies. In these situations, it is typical for doctors in our current healthcare system to hear such concerns and then rapidly offer only a prescription medicine. Many other avenues of care may work better, based on the individual and an understanding of their needs.

When we hold onto past emotional hurts or abuses caused by others, we are allowing that person or people to keep hurting us. Such forgiveness doesn't lessen the wrongdoing we experienced or the pain it caused us, but it does allow us to complete the experience and move forward more positively in our life. As with deeper issues or changing behaviors, it is easier said than done. This can be aided by inner work, delving into the subconscious and creating positive affirmations. This is really at the core of preventive medicine and improving health.

It is most often helpful to focus more upon our present and our future rather than on being held back by our past. Part of wholism (all of our dimensions) and integrative medicine is about healing transformation—moving from where we are to where we wish to be. Often, what we believe is what we perceive and receive from our surroundings, other people and the universe. Supporting our body, correcting and guiding our mind in the thinking we do and what we tell ourselves, and caring for our heart and emotions are all extremely important for healing and overall wellbeing.

Counseling and lifestyle coaching, which look at and help us with our stress levels and emotional issues, are important areas to explore, and an important part of education and preventive medicine. This is especially true in creating and maintaining healthy relationships with our loved ones, at home and at work, and making wiser and healthier choices. There are also many recovery programs for dealing with specific substance abuse issues, from food and alcohol, to nicotine and narcotic drugs. **I am an advocate of counseling and psychotherapy to avoid being "comfortably comfortable" with our accepted health-undermining habits,** which are not just food and substances but our overall behaviors. It does take a desire and practice, often with the help or support of others, to make positive changes and lessen the comforting habits. When we challenge ourselves, or have someone ask us deeper questions, or get involved in relationships that routinely challenge our concepts, behaviors and boundaries, we have a greater potential for awareness, change and growth. Identifying our issues is always a good start. Using the subconscious to create new healthy cellular memories and pathways helps to avoid repeat behaviors and supports new healthier ones. This is the basis of Hypnotherapy.

I encourage us all to embrace the underlying causes as to why we undermine our health with basically unwise choices and habits; it often lies in our self-image and attitudes toward self. Therapy and dealing with our emotional and psychological selves is often the beginning for positive change in our lives. Many find help with using positive affirmations and meditation to help them heal and feel better about themselves. The deepest level of health care and healing is to understand the emotional and psycho-spiritual issues that lie within the energies of dis-ease, and to reconnect with this human inter-dimensional de-synchrony, which includes healing the inherent conflicts within us. As stated in the conclusion of *Staying Healthy with the Seasons,*

"Illness is conflict and resistance to change; healing is growth and evolution. When we learn how to listen to the guidance within our being, within our psyche, and with an open aware-ness, where we embrace growth and change, we HEAL."

SPIRITUAL HEALING

What does this mean and what therapies are included? Prayer, meditation, energy transfer, distance healing are some examples of this topic. The dictionary definition states that *spiritual healing* uses practices such as prayer to make a person healthy. However, more modern approaches look at the perspective that an individ-ual could have an illness and still be spiritually healthy—meaning they have found purpose, love, connection to nature or a higher force, such as God.

Spiritual healing is not faith healing; its premise is that when we are more aligned with the larger universe, our purpose in life, our mind and body, we are healing ourselves spiritually. This is con-sidered by some to be part of life's journey. Specifically it involves energy. It is likely the most ancient form of medicine - shamanic healing could be considered spiritual as can going to church, working in a food bank, giving back, and/or being in a state of gratitude. This is an important part of a healthy lifestyle and can be tapped into through meditation.

"True is true, always and all ways. No matter what we say or do, true is true."
                                                                —ARGISLE

NEW MEDICINE CASE STUDY - INSOMNIA

Let's meet Jill, aged 49, who is in menopause transition experiencing some sweats and anxiety, as well as problems sleeping, which causes fatigue and even exhaustion.

Where do we start? It's quick and easy to give her Western drugs for sleep (such as Ambien or Sonata) and anxiety (Ativan or Xanax which also help for sleep), and even some estrogen to calm her hot flashes. Yet with NEW Medicine, we always want to look at the causes, which are partly her life changes, but also Jill's use of caffeine to get through her work day and alcohol to relax at night. Often however, this attempt at balance using stimulants and sedatives leads to being wired and tired, as Jill clearly was.

To begin with, we didn't want to start with hormone therapy, even bio-identical treatment, but Jill was willing to shift her diet and take a break from caffeine and alcohol. Instead we used good nutrition to help her transition and improve her daily energy with nutritious smoothies containing greens like chlorella and barley grass and a red high antioxidant powder that contains blueberry, acai, and pomegranate as examples. These morning drinks provided her energy that was more lasting than coffee and helped her calm down as well.

Jill also took GABA with L-Theanine and 5-hydroxytryptophan for calming at night and better sleep. With these improvements, her daily energy and attitude began to improve greatly, and her hot flashes lessened with better nutrition and acupuncture.

She had several acupuncture treatments, which were deeply relaxing during and energizing afterwards. Acupuncture is often helpful for anxiety and poor sleep as well. In addition, some Chinese herbs were used to go along with her other supplements, and included Suan Zao Ren San (for trouble falling asleep) and Tian Wang Bu Xing San (taken if awakened).

Jill was also given a low-dose Xanax (alprazolam) to use only if she couldn't sleep, or for a night when she had slept poorly the night before. She did take it a few times and she felt it helped to reset her sleep clock.

Jill felt better within a month, had improved energy, lost 7 pounds and felt much more positive about her life.

INSOMNIA CASE SUMMARY

- **Natural**—Lifestyle shifts with dietary and detox program, reducing stimulants, lowering EMF exposures, and using appropriate Natural Supplements and Herbs, such as GABA and Melatonin, Valerian root and Linden flowers

- **Eastern**—Balance energy to lessen excitability and agitation, and acupuncture treatments can be very calming, plus the use of specific Chinese Herbs.

- **Western**—Sedate the brain and nervous system with medications, tranquilizers and sleeping pills

When the pros and cons, the strengths and weaknesses, of each medical modality are understood, then we can choose the best treatment and the best time to apply it. Ultimately, the most appropriate of all available therapies and medicines are used together and integrated into a NEW Medicine approach for each person as a unique individual.

REVIEWING THE NEW MEDICINE APPROACH
Bringing Health back into Health Care

The intent of NEW Medicine is to guide each of you to become more aware and self-sufficient in your self care, your lifestyle, and when necessary to be your own best doctor, or primary care provider, using the healthcare system for your benefit, while learning and living in ways to avoid becoming a "patient" in the first place.

We are fortunate to live in a time when there are many good choices to consider and utilize, depending on what kinds of health challenges we are faced with in our life. Yet, this help typically costs time, energy and money, and to many it matters who is paying. The spectrum of options ranges from ancient, time-tested approaches to the most modern, cutting edge technologies. For example, with an auto accident or injuries from a fall, X-rays and pain medicines may be needed. We may also want to look at structural assessment and treatment to correct and rebalance the body. Osteopathy and structural care can help realign the skeleton; massage can help reduce muscle tightness as can simple stretching, breathing, and relaxing, and acupuncture can help to rebalance the meridians and our body's energy system.

NEW Medicine presents a uniquely integrated approach to our personal health as well as our healthcare system's problems, offering more HEALTH CARE and less disease care. It merges modern Western technologies of physical evaluation (such as lab tests and x-rays) with Natural and Eastern medicine approaches to assess health conditions and provide a combination of therapies that create a balanced and cost-effective approach to optimal health.

The three primary health systems of NEW Medicine represent an integration that alters our view of disease and offers the promise of sustainable health for us as individuals and as a society.

Of course, no one discipline of health care has all the answers. We each begin with where we are in our overall health and our lifestyle. Many of us try to get away with over-consumption and stressful lives until it's clear that we must change in order to feel better and survive. When more natural approaches can work, we apply those first unless we are acutely ill and need immediate intervention, which is where Western medicine is often so helpful. Many practitioners and patients, especially those that have studied several healing systems, believe this to be the case. We start by addressing causes and then in regard to treatment, we think:

> *"Lifestyle First,*
> *Natural Therapies Next,*
> *Drugs or Western Medical Intervention Last."*

We have talked about *patient or personal responsibility*, but what about doctor responsibility? It clearly makes sense that to be a good doctor, we need to know about all the systems of health care that our patients are using, especially nowadays with the internet and a more educated population. Remember, the word "doctor" comes from the Latin word *docere*, which means "teach," and it is a physician's key role to teach her or his patients about the ways of the body and the ways to health. Frankly, we have lost that original definition in Western conventional, drug-based medicine, but not in the Traditional Medicine practices of Naturopathy, Eastern Medicine, Acupuncture and even Chiropractic.

First of course, the doctors much teach themselves. When I changed my diet choices and eating habits, it made a huge difference in my health, and doing regular cleansing and detoxification programs has made an even more significant impression. Because of my experience, I have been able to inspire and guide thousands of people over the years in this positive healing process, as well as remain in better health myself on an ongoing basis.

I did my first cleansing fast in 1975 and it altered my health in amazing ways. "This is the only body I have, and I am going to treat it with love," is what I told myself. With this overall attitude shift, I began to eat better, exercise and stretch my body, and take care of myself emotionally and spiritually, and thus be open to learn and grow. This is what I have been asking my patients and audiences to do over these past 40 years, and I see this as one of the most important messages in health care.

MOTIVATION IS KEY

The critical question is: **How do we motivate people to care for themselves?** Only a few things motivate most people. My associate, Bethany Argisle, told me many decades ago, "People change from crisis or vanity." In other words, you are falling apart, or you look (to yourself) like you're falling apart. Of course, some people make change for other reasons, such as an awakened desire to love their body or be healthier for themselves and family, or for scientific curiosity to see if certain changes provide improved results, as in less symptoms or greater energy and vitality. We must decide that our health is a good investment!

Often, it takes an upcoming wedding or school reunion for people to do the hard work to eat less, make better food choices, and give up some unhealthy favorites. Starting or enhancing an exercise program can also be a challenge. Even those of us who work out regularly can get complacent in their routines. If I get into a rut, I may enlist a trainer to work out with me, and they knowingly tell me how to improve, often with just a few adjustments.

Being or seeing good examples for healthy living is also motivating. Scare tactics with statistics and pictures of what might happen to people if they keep smoking or eating their poor diet is not as helpful as inspiration. Nor is blame or shame, or feeling guilty; we need to truly wish to seek optimal health. When I ask young people what would motivate them to take better care of themselves, they tell me to give them a picture or a sense of what would be better if they behaved in a different way. Some of us may be motivated by better looking skin or having more energy and better sexual function, but we could also be motivated to just feel better and have more vitality and love of life every day. Yet, most do not; it takes personal searching and focus to keep our motivation and goals alive.

Enlisting others to motivate and support us, challenge us, or exercise with us is often a valuable investment in our health. This is why my Detox Groups work well and people achieve their goals more easily with the support and camaraderie they experience. It may still be worth doing some consultation or treatment if it brings about change and improves our health, although this care may not be covered by insurance. Friends' help is free and they can support us to stay motivated as well. Some of the other services that can be helpful might involve structural care and massage, acupuncture, or seeing a counselor/therapist, and often on a consistent basis to simply be well.

Of course, pain and suffering or an incident like a heart attack scare are often the dominant factors that motivate most people towards improved care and to change their state of health. Money is of course also a major consideration, yet good health, and staying out of the riskier and potentially expensive therapies of Western medicine is important to many; to the wise, health is more important than "mere money."

Many natural practitioner's services are not covered by insurance and must be paid for out-of-pocket, yet many people actually spend less time and money dealing with illness and medical problems when they maintain their health and live more naturally. At my clinic, I incorporate the New Medicine principles and practices into insurance-based healthcare delivery on a daily basis, and have experienced first hand--and therefore believe--that this approach offers a significant improvement in overall care, results and costs. **This approach needs to be studied further and then supported throughout our entire healthcare system by the government's allocation of dollars and resources for prevention, education and proactive protection of our people's health, including the safety of our environment.**

In contrast to a Western Medicine approach, the core of Natural and Eastern Medicines, thus NEW Medicine, is **prevention and treating the underlying causes of disease**—helping people understand what's out of balance and what can be changed, ideally before disease reaches a crisis stage. It's not always up to doctors and their staff, or even the healthcare system. Fundamentally it's up to each of us!

"To Heal, we must take time for Health."   —ARGISLE

94

THE KEY MESSAGES OF NEW MEDICINE

For Patients and Students

- Take responsibility for preventing illness through healthy lifestyle choices

- Understand and address illnesses more effectively and earlier whenever they occur

- Use an intelligent blend of natural approaches, ancient wisdom, and evidence-based technology of modern medicine

For Doctors and Practitioners

- Focus on the "whole person" and overall health patterns, and not just symptoms

- Move from seeing patients to seeing "people" patiently

- Recognize that healing is first and foremost an internal process, not one that is always addressed with external drugs and surgery

- Educate your patients to help maintain health and prevent disease

- Investigate the various Natural, Eastern and Western therapies to incorporate new insights and complementary treatment options for common health problems into your practice.

For Everyone

- Live life fully and keep Love in your Heart

- Make every day count

- By adding more life to your days, you may also be adding more days to your life.

CHAPTER 2

NEW MEDICINE PRINCIPLES
Understanding Causes

To continue the quote from the introduction:

"Wise people should consider that health is their most valuable possession, and learn how by their own thoughts to derive benefit from illness."

—HIPPOCRATES

IN THE INTRODUCTION and first chapter, we have explored ideas for resolving some of the problems in our healthcare system using an integrated NEW Medicine approach. We suggested a new focus on **educating people to take personal responsibility and appropriate steps to live well, prevent disease, and develop a collaborative relationship between patients and health-care providers to create the greatest benefits at the lowest possible cost**. This is a big goal to consider. This broad approach requires each individual to be more responsible for his or her health instead of relying solely on the doctor or the system to provide a so-called cure for every illness or health concern. Timely support-ive follow-up care is essential and should be a shared by all con-cerned—for patients, their families, and practitioners alike—and an emphasis on early education about Staying Healthy.

Focus on three primary areas of lifestyle
**NUTRITION
EXERCISE
& STRESS**
can improve health outcomes.

Staying Healthy with NEW Medicine is especially relevant as our population ages, when health needs often increase and we experience a desire to improve our wellbeing and vitality—what we might term *Healthy Aging.* Also, NEW Medicine looks at, and aligns with, how our health choices affect the envi-ronmental challenges facing this precious planet.

The first approach that makes a difference for my patients is to explain and demonstrate to them how to adapt their lifestyles in three key areas of health—eating better, exercising more, and man-aging their stress.[1] By improving these areas, a person's health most often improves, with fewer breakdowns, requiring less costly crises and interventions.

Research shows that focusing on these three key areas can be effec-tive in reducing the incidence and cost of many chronic problems, including Obesity and Diabetes, as well as Cardiovascular Disease and Cancer.[2] Yet, it's not information, or knowing something is good or bad for us that is the primary motivation to change behavior or habits; it's an internal decision made by each individual. Sometimes, changes are encouraged by a crisis, such as a heart attack scare, or from vanity, where we just awaken to the idea that our body is aging or breaking down. Of course, wanting to look better and feel better helps with this decision to improve lifestyle.[3]

CHANGING HABITS = IMPROVED HEALTH

One example of a low-cost phone-based intervention was explored with a poor urban population in the San Francisco Bay Area. Contacted by phone about once a month, half of the 230 people in the study received specific dietary guidance and lifestyle counseling. After six months, those who had received education and counseling had on average lost more weight, were consuming less fat, were eating more fruits and vegetables, and showed more improvements in lowering in their blood triglycerides, a key risk measure for type 2 diabetes.[4]

The US Center for Disease Control and Prevention estimates that eliminating three risk factors—poor diet, inactivity, and smoking—would prevent 80% of heart disease,[5] stroke, and type 2 diabetes, plus 40% of cancer.[6]

Prevention begins with education and community-based programs that help turn around the current crises of a growing number of people with chronic yet preventable diseases. Although increasing, funding at a national level has been limited; therefore, individual health care providers and patients MUST do their part.

THE GOAL OF NEW MEDICINE

An integrative, health-oriented educational approach provides guidance for people to correct causes of ill health beforehand and to create healthier lifestyles. Ultimately, our health maintenance is up to each of us through our daily choices, along with utilizing, when necessary, healthcare providers to guide, teach and treat us when appropriate. One of my maxims is: **"Better choices create better health outcomes."** Yet, as you know, there are many types of choices—not only about food and drugs, but also relationships and attitudes—all are crucial aspects of our lives.

How's your Lifestyle?

Take a few moments to reflect on these questions related to your way of life:

- Are you currently doing anything or everything to promote your optimal health?
- Are there areas where you can do better. Stress, diet or exercise, social support?
- What changes are you making now?
- Do you take personal responsibility for your health or are you willing to.
- What about those in your family; how are they doing?
- Have you given up any health-undermining habits?
- Do you trust or mistrust life?
- Do you expect it to treat you badly or well?
- Do you have an underlying attitude of loving yourself, so that you can maintain good habits to support your body and health?
- If not, are you interested in changing your attitude?
- Are you stuck in the past?
- Do you fear the future?
- What happens if you do "everything right" and still encounter health challenges? How will you handle that?

These and similar questions highlight a few of the layers in looking at our health challenges. Remember, "Health is our greatest Wealth." You only have one body per life and who's going to care for it if you don't?

THE UNDERLYING PRINCIPLES OF NEW MEDICINE

When changing and improving the way we approach our personal health care, it is essential that our basic underlying philosophy about health and healing works for us. Also, for any effective healthcare practice to claim improved outcomes with patients, there must be a demonstrable reduction in medical problems and a significant improvement in patients making meaningful differences in their health and quality of life.

Every day in my practice I see improvements such as lowered risk factors and costs when people make lifestyle changes including stopping smoking, losing weight, changing their diet and managing stress.[7, 8] Of course, lowering healthcare costs is also a goal. I have learned over the decades that the most effective philosophy to facilitate change is when I am aligned with my patient's belief. When we believe our choices will help us feel better, we are more likely to take action. And when our health providers are optimistic with us, change can happen more readily.

There are a few essential questions to ask when trying to explore your own beliefs about health and illness:

- What are the underlying causes of illness?
- What can you do to prevent illness and enhance prevention?
- How do you treat an illness or injury when it does occur?
- Who has supported your health, and who, or what, has not?

WHAT IS HEALTH AND HEALING?

Before we look at the causes of illness in the body, let's explore the idea and definition of Health and then ask, **"What is true healing?"** The World Health Organization (WHO) defines health as "a state of complete physical, mental and social wellbeing and not merely the absence of disease or infirmity." **True healing often means going far deeper than treating the physical symptoms of disease or poor health. It involves looking at the underlying causes, and sensing the nature of the changes that a person needs to make to eliminate a health problem, to prevent disease and to optimize wellbeing.** There are many sources of healing—they can be in our personal life path choices, in our relationships, in our spiritual connections, our emotional resilience, how we manage stresses or other mental/emotional conflicts. Also, of course, they include our diet, our level of physical activity, amount and consistency of stress, and in the way we use or abuse certain substances, plus what we inherit from our genetics and family upbringing.

"Health is a vital state of functional activity with all body systems working optimally together, including the physical body with the mind, emotions and spirit to support our vitality and life force. In this state, we have fewer risks and episodes of disease, imbalance, and health complaints. We can then maintain a sense of wellbeing more easily, which is a consequence of a healthy lifestyle, attitude, and peace of mind."
—DR. ELSON

102

HEALING

Our bodies, minds, and emotions—and our overall health—are all constantly changing. The need to heal is not just when we experience a specific illness or symptom—rather it is part of a sustainable healthy process that goes on all the time. We are always learning, growing and healing.

Healing also comes from insight into areas of personal conflict; the relief of stress and struggle; the lessening of tension and pessimism: the reduction of inflammation; the eradication of infectious agents that undermine the body's function; the replenishment of depleted nutrients; and the continued nourishment of body, mind, heart and spirit.

There are also spiritual aspects of healing that may be separate from the experience of physical problems or diseases. We can experience healing at emotional and energetic levels, while our body may still have some medical issues. We might consider that there are two different tracks or paths in the body—one for medical treatment and another for healthy living.

Our primary goal is living well and feeling good on an ongoing basis. Medically speaking, preventing disease is a primary goal—if we don't get sick in the first place, are we are already "healed?" What if we carry the genetic potential for any disease, yet feel fine--are we still healthy, and if so, until when? From my experience, there is a wide spectrum that ranges from illness, to not being sick, to being actively healthy and vital. Or we could look at healing as merely a reduction or elimination of symptoms and disease. If we take something that helps our headache get better, is that healing? Many would say yes; others, no. We could bring together a hundred great medical minds, even thousands, and it is unlikely that we could come up with a definition of health, or healing, that all would embrace. I encourage you to consider your own definitions based on the principles of NEW Medicine, so we can begin to look at health and healing in a new and expanded way.

The Health Continuum

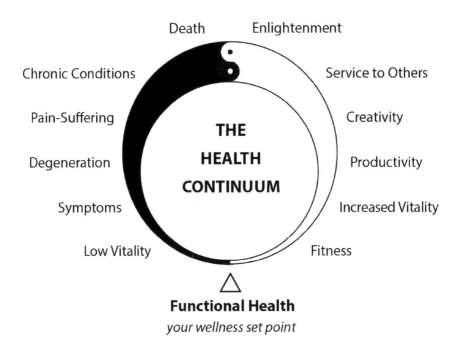

Death   Enlightenment

Chronic Conditions   Service to Others

Pain-Suffering   Creativity

Degeneration   **THE HEALTH CONTINUUM**   Productivity

Symptoms   Increased Vitality

Low Vitality   Fitness

Functional Health
your wellness set point

Most of us settle at some wellness set point and wait to get sick—then we work to heal and return to our former state. But what about optimizing our health and enhancing our energy, fitness and vitality? Of course, the stages of the continuum are not mutually exclusive—you can be sick and in pain and still be creative and serving others; you can also be healthy and vital and not productive or caring about others or our planet. However, as we move towards greater health and vitality, we are more able to activate these higher qualities of life.

DEFINITIONS OF HEALTH

Hippocrates suggested that, "Health is the expression of the harmonious balance of various aspects of a human's nature, environment, and ways of living." Does that sound as though one of the founders of Medicine thought health was related to our lifestyle?

World Health Organization: "Health is the complete physical, mental, and sociological well-being, not just the absence of disease or infirmity."

OrthoMolecular Health/Medicine Society - a legacy of the late Linus Pauling: "Health is the result of having all the right molecules in the right amounts in the right places." (*This ties into the idea of cellular health, deficiency and toxicity discussed later in this chapter.*)

Dr. Elson: "Health is a sense of well-being that incorporates function and environment, awareness and vitality, productivity and peace. Ultimately, it is the outcome of the alignment of body, mind, heart and spirit, and the connection with the path that lives at the core of our being."

Tara West: "Feeling vibrant and vital, flexible and strong, and passionate about each day's work and play. That's good health to me."

What Is Your Definition of Health? What's important to you?

I believe in and practice a simple common sense philosophy about health and health care—*how we look and feel is primarily the result of how we live;* if we want a different result, how we live must change. **When seeking to sort out the causative factors of ill health, all behaviors become suspect and most are testable, meaning we evaluate them by avoiding them for a period of time,**

**look at results, and then assess any reactions by re-intro-
ducing them into our lives.** These issues include regular substance usage as with caffeine and alcohol or sugar habits, food
choices (based on knowledge, balance, understanding food labels,
if we can see the fine print) and other lifestyle activities such as
sleep, exercise, rest and relaxation, and handling emotional and
environmental stresses. Of course, it's not just about eliminating
something, but also adding healthy behaviors such as eating more
fresh vegetables, getting regular exercise and stretching, and reducing stress. Ideally, we can focus much more on healing and improving life and vitality, than on what's wrong and trying to fix that with
the latest treatment.

"Energy is the gold; we spend it on our life, and we are the outcome."

—ARGISLE

Most of us are blessed with fairly good health as youngsters, yet, by
the time we are in our teens, or even pre-teens, many begin to experience declining health as now evidenced by the epidemic of childhood obesity in many developed countries. For those of us who are
already grown, this education, or really re-education, about what it
takes to support our healthy human body happens not only in our
homes and schools, but also at our doctor's office during routine
checkups or medical visits, or as special classes supported by the
practice or community. Realize that the media has a much greater
influence on our health and habits than ever before, not only due to
the number and size of media advertisers, but due to the expanding
array of technologies and methods for delivering messages.

WHAT CAUSES ILL HEALTH AND DISEASE?

Having defined what we mean by health and healing, let's now explore the NEW Medicine understanding of what causes disease. Life is multidimensional; so, often the causes of illness and disease are not simple, linear, cause-and-effect interactions. Disease typically arises from a field of complex interactions between our genetic make-up and the entirety of our life circumstances, which includes personal lifestyle factors such as the quality of diet, exercise and stress levels as well as external environmental factors such as microbes, chemicals and toxins in our air, water, food, home and workplace.

Stress, for example, can be the result of disease as well as a contributor to many problems. Lack of exercise, physical fitness and flexibility can result in weight issues and low vitality, while being overweight or having low motivation may cause us to avoid exercise. Plus, we can become injured with too much exercise, or overdoing it, especially when we are not in shape. Overall, Western Medicine is a linear system, while the Eastern and Natural Medicine disciplines are more integrative in general. This is why a multidisciplinary integrated approach is so important and useful in addressing health issues more completely. Let's look deeper at what is believed about causes of illness.

When people are sick, what is at the core of their illness? Is it a germ that some friend had and passed on? Isn't there always something going around? Why do some people experience high levels of health while others seem to be perpetually suffering from one health problem or another? There are often identifiable causal agents for specific illnesses, but even still, all illnesses are multi-factorial and often mysterious to sort out. Beyond the specific causes of illness, there is a broader philosophy of the many underlying layers of disease-causing factors that may be viewed from the integrated approach of NEW Medicine and the real CAUSES of disease.

SYMPTOMS AND ILLNESSES AS SIGNS OF HEALING OR IMBALANCE

Often, what we experience as symptoms is actually the body's attempt to heal itself. This is a naturopathic principle that relates to detoxification and "healing crises." We know this in regard to fever, which many people interpret as something wrong and then take aspirin to lower it. However, now many are beginning to understand that the increase in body temperature has beneficial effects to help fight infection, kill microbes, and enhance immune defenses. When experiencing colds, sinus congestion, or skin rashes, one natural health interpretation is that the body is trying to clear itself of "toxins" and ideally should not be suppressed. When we suppress symptoms, we disrupt the natural elimination of congestion or toxicity; and although we may reduce our external symptoms, we are not truly healed. We're actually slowing down the body's healing process.

Some symptoms that fall into this category as expressions of imbalance, toxicity, and the body's attempt to detoxify include: headaches, the itchiness of allergies, runny nose and sinus congestion; general aches and pains; skin rashes; and diarrhea and digestive upset. When issues like these arise, we want to understand where they come from (and why), make appropriate adjustments and adapt in ways that can help us resolve them.

PRIMARY CAUSES AND FACTORS UNDERLYING DISEASE

- **CELL HEALTH**

  Deficiency and Toxicity

- **GENETICS AND EPIGENETICS**

- **LIFESTYLE**

  Family Patterns and Upbringing

  Nutrition

  Exercise

  Stress

- **EXTERNAL ENVIRONMENT**

CELL HEALTH

Health is based on the physical and energetic needs of our cells to thrive. If we look at these requirements it becomes easier to understand why certain activities influence our health. Remember, our body is made of trillions of our own cells and ten times more that are bacteria living in harmony with us, mainly in our gut.

Each body cell functions on its own and as part of the whole. Also, each one has particular functions that are important to the entire body operating optimally. Each activity within cells—whether it's to make more hormones, engage a dangerous invader, or get rid of dead or dangerous materials—requires energy. So the cellular energy-making apparatus must be efficient, well watered and fed with required nutrients, and given lots of good clean air/oxygen.

A NOTE ON CAUSES

The attempt to develop a linear model of causes is challenging given our non-linear world. Life can be complex and everything does not have one simple causative factor. For example, with low thyroid function, fatigue and weight gain, there may be many issues at play, including genetics, infections, malfunction or immune attack on the thyroid, diet imbalances, and stress. Similarly a heart attack is often the culmination of decades of poor diet, genetic predisposition, stress, and other factors. And what about the person whose lifestyle is ideal, but still gets a heart attack or cancer? How do we explain that?

We need some points of entry and understanding to elucidate the deeper factors underlying any disease process. Given that Western medical research generally has a more linear view of the causes and effects of disease, and Eastern and Natural Medicines may be more non-linear, it makes sense to integrate their best aspects. I am also aware that I could discuss this topic with many brilliant scientists and thinkers and we would not agree on all of the concepts and connections I propose. However, I think numerous practitioners and healers of all systems of medicine would concur with many of these ideas.

The outer circle of the chart labeled **"Outcomes"** shows common symptoms and medical problems. These are typical of what WM doctors treat, usually with an outside-in approach involving symptom suppression. *In NEW Medicine we are suggesting an inside-out orientation,* going deeper to understand and address underlying causes. Heal the "insides," or lifestyle, and many of the outcomes will improve. Most people and their physicians are satisfied simply to name the diseases and offer medicines to reduce the symptoms or lower the numbers, such as blood sugar, blood pressure, or cholesterol. This is not real healing. I suggest that while treating symptoms and numbers, we also work to address and correct primary and secondary causes.

CAUSES OF DISEASE
THE NEW MEDICINE MODEL

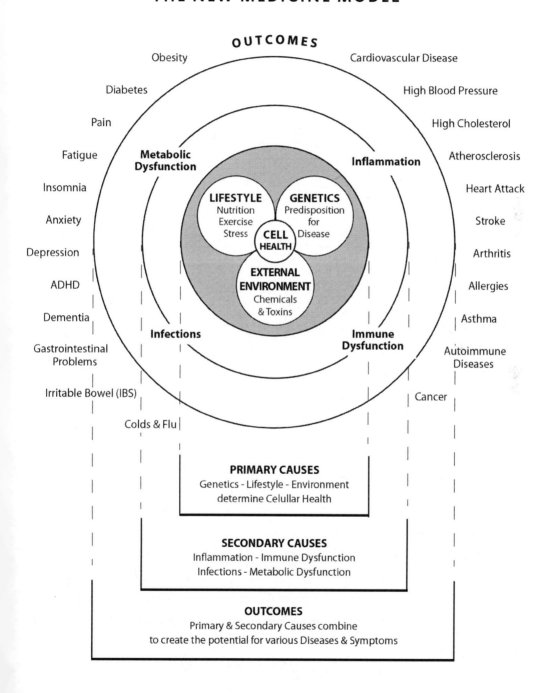

OUTCOMES

Obesity   Cardiovascular Disease

Diabetes   High Blood Pressure

Pain   High Cholesterol

Fatigue   **Metabolic Dysfunction**   **Inflammation**   Atherosclerosis

Insomnia   Heart Attack

Anxiety   **LIFESTYLE** Nutrition Exercise Stress   **GENETICS** Predisposition for Disease   Stroke

CELL HEALTH

Depression   Arthritis

ADHD   **EXTERNAL ENVIRONMENT** Chemicals & Toxins   Allergies

Dementia   Asthma

Gastrointestinal Problems   **Infections**   **Immune Dysfunction**   Autoimmune Diseases

Irritable Bowel (IBS)   Cancer

Colds & Flu

PRIMARY CAUSES
Genetics - Lifestyle - Environment
determine Celullar Health

SECONDARY CAUSES
Inflammation - Immune Dysfunction
Infections - Metabolic Dysfunction

OUTCOMES
Primary & Secondary Causes combine
to create the potential for various Diseases & Symptoms

Energy depletion usually comes from stress and insufficient nutrition and may result in *cellular malfunction* that can be the route to many ailments in the body—from a bad mood, to poor thinking, to experiencing recurrent infections. The mitochondria are the parts of our cells that convert food to energy and are most at danger from toxic free radicals (unstable molecules that can inflame the body). **This process is a classic example of how what we eat and how we manage stress both may play a big role in keeping our cells and our entirety well fueled and protected from damage.**

DEFICIENCY AND TOXICITY

When talking about cell nutrition, let's consider the many nutrients we need—vitamins, minerals, amino acids (proteins), fatty acids, glucose and phytonutrients—which are essential for our cells and tissues to function optimally. Our cells perform countless activities daily, and consistently require specific nutrients to work properly. I list some of these in the upcoming section on Nutrition.

Nutrient deficiencies can diminish cellular functions, while toxicities from environmental chemicals (and metals like lead and mercury) in our air, water and food can undermine or poison cellular functions, by damaging enzymes and even causing mutations in our DNA. Thousands of enzymes are crucial proteins that catalyze (or speed up) metabolic reactions, allowing cell activities to go along smoothly. Stress and deficiencies can also cause oxidative damage to cells and tissues and contribute to inflammation.

Cells must be able to accurately decipher and translate genetic instructions so we must do what we can to protect our genes from damaging toxins, radiation, and stress to maintain their healthy expressions. For example, one way to protect the genes in our skin cells is to stay out of the intense sun mid-day; this may lessen the risk and incidence of skin cancers. Another way to protect cells from oxidative stress is to make sure you have a diet rich in antioxidant foods like tomatoes and watermelon that are rich in lycopene; nuts and seeds with selenium, zinc, and other minerals; and many fruits and vegetables that contain B vitamins, C, and minerals.

Damage to our cells can create a variety of cell dysfunctions and then the energy-producing mitochondria can become less active, resulting in less energy for your cells and body to do its work and repair. Damage can come from internal breakdowns or external assaults, microbial attacks and nutrient deficiencies.

Taking care of our cells means taking care of ourselves in body, heart and mind. How we think, what we believe—in other words, our attitudes—influence our actions. Our behaviors and choices (be they healthy or unhealthy) contribute to/determine whether we are healthy, happy, worn down or sick.

"One mouth or another; which one this time? We eat sounds, smells, and sights, plus thoughts and feelings—not only foods." —ARGISLE

The bottom line is that cellular dysfunction is one of the primary causes of body imbalance, inflammation, and disease. Cellular functions are what keep us alive and well. When we exercise or meditate, we fill our cells with life-giving oxygen. When we worry, we flood our cells and tissues with stress chemicals. And when we experience pleasure, we flood them with pain-diminishing molecules. Cells R Us![9]

GENETICS

Our inherited genetic makeup influences our basic nature, constitutional state of health, and potential for certain risk factors and health problems. Most often however, unless we have problematic genetic errors, our health is damaged primarily by our own actions and habits, both personally and in our environment. Ultimately our lifestyle and daily activities are the main contributing factors that lead us to stay healthy or not—those factors and areas of life over which we have control. As I like to say, *"Much of our health is up to each of us."*

EPIGENETICS

Also, how our lifestyle habits and choices influence what problems we develop or don't develop is beginning to be explored in a new field called *Epigenetics*. This is the study of how the expression of our genes is affected by diet, exercise, and lifestyle, and even our ancestors' lifestyles.Early research shows that our choices—whether we smoke, the foods we eat, and any nutrient deficiencies—can influence the expression of our genes, protecting us or putting us more at risk for certain diseases. Of course, this is still in the experimental mode, but just think of the potential of this groundbreaking discovery. The concept that how we live affects the outcome of our genetic potential is a great breakthrough!

So what you eat may not only affect your own genes, but also your grandchildren's health. Every cell in your body inherits genetic instructions from your parents. Yet, each cell uses those instructions differently due to the internal switches that turn certain information on or off.

EPIGENETICS: AN EXAMPLE FROM RESEARCH

The research that first exemplified this understanding of epigenetic influence was done with "fat, sickly yellow mice." These obese mice were gluttons and prone to cancer and diabetes. Scientists wanted to see if they could alter the health outcomes of these overeating, unhealthy mice. The cause of these problems was in the genes, specifically the "agouti gene". In the study, before the mice became pregnant, they were fed a better diet with certain supplements (namely folic acid, vitamin B12, and methionine), and their babies were born slender, with their natural brown color, and without the devastating life-threatening illnesses of their mothers. They stayed healthy and lived longer. They still had the 'bad gene,' but the dietary changes for the mother rendered the babies' "agouti" gene 'silent.' These dietary induced epigenetic changes were inherited through several generations of mice.[10]

Unfortunately, we don't yet know how to reliably turn off the genes that may contribute to human illness. However, groundbreaking studies from Dr. Dean Ornish with men with prostate cancer, showed that when they changed their lifestyle for three months—eating a vegetarian diet, exercising, medititating and participating in group support—the expression of their prostate cancer genes was lessened while their protective genes were expressed more strongly.[11]

This information suggests that **our daily actions, what we eat, how much we consume, and if we smoke, not only affect us directly, but can also affect the health of our children, grandchildren and even their children.** Lifestyle makes a big difference not only in our own health but possibly in that of future generations.

PREDISPOSITION FOR DISEASE

People are typically susceptible to certain diseases such as heart disease, cancer, colitis, arthritis, allergies or asthma due to their genetics, family patterns and upbringing, Our past influences our present lifestyle behaviors, which over time, can lead to health problems that we must handle. Many risk factors can be detected in early exams and blood tests, such as a poor cholesterol/HDL ratio and other aspects of lipid profiles and cholesterol readings. So an important aspect of Preventive Medicine is to identify specific individual risk factors in order to be proactive in changing habits that could be contributing to or exacerbating a problem; this can make a real difference to our health in the long run. Being proactive could means paying attention to how dietary fats and sugars affect our cholesterol levels and our risk for cardiovascular problems, or knowing that our sugar intake and excess weight are risks for developing type-2 diabetes. These serious and prevalent illnesses are linked to high-sugar diets and the intake of "bad" and poorly utilized fats that can cause inflammation. We also know that certain habits like cigarette smoking are risk factors for many diseases, and become an expense for us all. It is therefore important to recognize how our unique genetic propensity, our environment, and our lifestyle patterns all contribute—for better or worse—to our overall health and wellness. The key is to know what we can control, what can be changed, and then do what we can to live the healing process in a **committed relationship to our health**.

LIFESTYLE: FAMILY PATTERNS AND UPBRINGING

Many of our choices and habits (good and bad) begin in our childhood with the ways our family lives—what and how we eat, how we relate emotionally, our family dynamics, and how physically active our parents are. These conditions and behaviors can create challenges in our own habits and motivations, yet we can change them throughout our lifetime to improve our health, so each of us can develop similar, different, or none of the problems that run in our families. The effects of family patterns and upbringing are influential, albeit to a lesser degree than our genetics; yet, over time, they may trump our genetic predisposition for disease. Our childhood patterns can be physical if we had a poor diet and became overweight, or they can be psychological—affecting our emotional behaviors and attitudes toward self and others, which then affect how we care for ourselves. Of course, our patterns are all encompassing in how we live each day. Is it in a loving or a hostile and abusive environment, with a rich or poor family, eating fast food or fresh foods? Clearly, when we grow up in a family with two loving and caring parents, who are at least somewhat conscious about health, it gives us a much better start and base for our own good health. Sadly, this is not always the case in families today.

As children, our parents and society at large have a far greater influence over our environment, our diet, and the choices we can make about our health, including our ideas and attitudes about life and the habits we develop in relation to food, stress, emotional behavior, etc. Ideally, these influences are blessings; for others, we spend much of our life getting over or correcting the misinformation or poor lifestyle habits imposed upon us (often unwittingly) in terms of physical, mental and emotional ways of being.

HEALING OUR INNER CHILD

Growing up, we all had some form of parenting, be it two long-term, loving parents, or angry frustrated people who fought and divorced when we were young. Some parents were kind and supportive; others were abusive and mean. Some were happy with their lives; others were not. No matter what, each parent talked to us in certain ways, and influenced us emotionally and physically, both positively and negatively. If we were loved and believed in with some level of accolade, or we did well in school or sports, ideally we began to develop our self-confidence that we were unique and valued by those around us. Let's face it, no matter how good things were, most of us have had issues around healing our parental and family patterns to become a strong individualized self and grow into healthy adulthood. Our family dynamic in terms of siblings also influenced how we evolved as responsible and caring adults, as well as how the greater world reflected life at home and community.

Facing the challenges and patterns of childhood, we can correct past misconceptions about our health, and then healing potential can improve with our intent and focus to be aware and more responsible.

- Where are you in the process of changing from your early negative exposures and experiences?
- What positive benefits do you experience from good influences?
- What seems to be the most important family behaviors to understand and change?

EXPLORING CHILDHOOD PATTERNS:
WHAT WAS IT LIKE FOR YOU?

- My parents were loving towards me.

- I could always depend on one parent to talk to.

- My parents were physically active and encouraged me to be the same.

- I lived in an abusive household.

- I was popular and liked.

- I had lots of friends.

- I loved school and learning.

- I did well in school.

- I was supportive of others.

- My family was always stressed about money.

- We shared at least one meal a day around the table.

- I shopped, cooked and ate with my family.

- Most meals were freshly cooked and well balanced.

- Most meals were fast food or prepackaged.

- We ate vegetables every day.

- I overeat.

- I eat while watching TV

- I eat too much late at night.

- We never had enough to eat.

- I was fat.

- I was skinny.

*How do such childhood issues, both positive and negative,
influence your behaviors today?*

One story about resolving the pain of parental family and self issues (for healing the "inner child"), comes from one of my favorite movies, Good Will Hunting, where Matt Damon plays a brilliant, yet emotionally damaged janitor at MIT. Robin Williams, playing his therapist, tells him in a very cathartic and healing interaction, "Will, it's not your fault." Repeatedly, "Will, it's not your fault" (that his father was an abusive and angry alcoholic who beat him). There is much violence, bitter divorce, and troubled behavior in the world, and children need to know, "It's not your fault."

LIFESTYLE: NUTRITION—EXERCISE—STRESS

These essential elements of health are explored more fully in The 5 Keys to Staying Healthy in the next chapter.

NUTRITION

As mentioned above, a primary cause for most disease is ***cellular dysfunction*** that arises from two main sources: **Deficiency**—not getting all the nutrients our body needs, and **Toxicity**—intake of and exposure to toxins that affect enzymes and cellular functions. (Of course, stress also affects cell function as well as our utilization of nutrients.) Our cells require literally thousands of molecules that are part of the foods we eat and the beverages we drink. These molecules provide much more than calories; they give us our vitamins and minerals, amino acids for protein, carbohydrates for energy, key essential fatty acids, cholesterol, many phytonutrients, etc. When bodies do not receive adequate supplies of high quality **essential nutrients**, the cells become deficient, which impairs function and can cause a decline in the health of tissues, organs and ultimately our entire body.

ESSENTIAL NUTRIENTS FOR AVOIDING DEFICIENCY

Macronutrients:

Proteins and amino acids, carbohydrates, fats and essential oils

Micronutrients:

Vitamins: A, C, D, E, K, B1, B6, B3, B12, CoQ10, Lipoic acid *(Most must come from our diet, and a few the body makes, like CoQ10 and lipoic.)*

Minerals: all must come from diet and include calcium, magnesium, potassium, sodium, zinc, copper, iron, manganese, selenium, iodine, traces of boron and others. *And our soil must contain these minerals to be in our food, and much soil is depleted.*

Phytonutrients: hundreds of plant substances, such as flavonoids and carotenoids, which give our fruits, vegetables, herbs and basically all foods their color, aroma, and add to their flavor.

Antioxidants: these nutrients protect us from "free radicals," the unstable molecules that can cause inflammation and damage; these nutrients include Vitamins A (and beta-carotene), C, D, and E plus some B vitamins; minerals zinc and selenium, with protective activity also from iron and magnesium; coenzyme Q10 and alpha lipoic acid; and amino acid L-cysteine, which helps support glutathione.

As discussed above we must also address **Toxicity**—the exposures of our cells to metals such as mercury or lead, smog, and cigarette smoke and damaging chemicals (e.g. pesticides, preservatives and cleaning agents) that come into our bodies from our air, water and foods. In addition, our cells create their own toxic chemicals, some of which are called oxidants or free radicals. Our cells have developed ways to remove these elements, but we need to provide them with appropriate antioxidants (vitamins C, A, E, and more) to facilitate the process of detoxification. We live in a world with many toxic elements in our consumer products. Even a cell that is well nourished can be adversely affected by exposure to such harmful substances.

EXERCISE

We need physical activity to keep our bodies fit and healthy. We stretch and move actively to maintain flexibility, to circulate our blood and lymph, to sweat and detoxify and to maintain a healthy weight, since most all of us love to eat. Basically, a regular exercise program helps relieve stress and includes stretching for flexibility, aerobics for endurance and cardiovascular fitness, and weight training for strength and bone/muscle building. And if you aren't now exercising regularly, have a physical exam, and then build your endurance at a healthy pace as you make your new exercise plan.

There's a catch-22 with exercise. When we get out of shape or hurt ourselves or feel depressed (or too busy), we slow down or stop exercising. And when we don't exercise and stay fit, we can become depressed and don't care, eat more, gain weight, and lack energy and vitality. Then, we are out of shape (so are our cells) and it becomes more difficult to begin and maintain your good, balanced fitness program. Just consider that when we don't feel like doing any kind of exercise, that's when we need to do it even more.

STRESS

A core factor of the NEW Medicine philosophy relates to how we manage stress and how it affects our health. One definition of stress is the perception that we don't have the resources to handle a problem, such as energy to handle the demands of family and work, or money to pay all the bills. Stress is created by how we handle our day-to-day lives and how we choose to act, react, or not act, in relation to our experiences.

Of course, **stress is a major contributing factor for disease or slower healing,** and it affects many levels of our being, including our cells, organs, our entire body and our minds. There are external stressors and internal ones. Our local environment provides many physical stressors, such as chemical toxins, electromagnetic exposures and intense weather activities. Mental stresses have to do with work, money, general attitudes and personal demands (and how they relate to our individual goals) while psycho-emotional stresses often correlate with relationship and family challenges. I believe that psycho-emotional stress, often caused by childhood and family patterns, can act as a primary cause of many health issues

---

"Is your health just another bill? Has your health lost its thrill?" —ARGISLE

We all start out with specific and unique genetics and then are influenced by our family's life and parents' patterns. These act as primary factors that lead to internal stresses, energy imbalances, intense emotions and often the choices we make later in life. For a variety of reasons, such as not feeling self-love, we may not treat ourselves in the best way with the best choices. In fact, we may be abusive or thoughtless with our personal habits, making poor food choices, smoking, drinking excessive alcohol or turning to drugs. Some of this may be based on genetics, yet most patterns and choices are rooted in our familial influence and training. How we were treated as children also affects our behaviors—physically, mentally, emotionally and in our hearts. When we suffer from abuse as children or young adults—or when we experience intense negative emotions of fear, shame or guilt (to name a few), this more easily leads to our personal abuse of self and others.

THE EXTERNAL ENVIRONMENT
CHEMICALS, TOXINS AND THEIR
CONNECTION TO OTHER PRIMARY CAUSES

The environment can have a significant impact on our health. It includes nutrition and the quality of what we choose to eat, the level of contaminants and toxins in foods we eat, the water we drink, the air we breathe and what we put on or around us. Clearly, everything in our lives affects our ability to function optimally and influences our overall healthy outcomes. Finding a balance and minimizing adverse environmental exposures helps us maintain our health. We are also surrounded and affected by allergens, smells and noise, electromagnetic pollution and what we see happening in the world, especially when we watch the nightly news! There are many things that we can alter to protect our selves from toxic assaults by our environment; yet, many exposures are inescapable, depending upon where we live. Be aware of this area of life - as always, all we can do is our best with what we know and believe.

In Beth Greer's informative book, *SuperNatural Home*, she divides external toxins into three categories: what we put IN us, ON us, and What Surrounds us. This is a helpful concept for looking at our lives and deciding where we can improve and lessen our toxin exposure.

Choose more natural, biodegradable products—at home, at work, in food propagation and preparation, and on our bodies—whenever and wherever possible. When living more naturally, we use fewer chemicals on and in our bodies and in our surroundings. This has a downstream effect—both over time and in our local environment. The goal to live more naturally involves a conscientious reduction in the use of synthetically made and petro-chemically-based products; plastics and petrol are a huge part of our modern existence. When we shop or travel around we are exposed to a wide variety of chemicals in stores, airports, planes, hotels, bathrooms, etc.

The shift to a more natural lifestyle and organic farming is growing across our nation and the globe, and is based largely on the same principles as *NEW Medicine:* taking personal responsibility for our health and for the planet, and recognizing the incredibly complex interactions between the decisions we make, the products we use, and their affect upon our entire environment and ecosystem, including our own health.

The effects of this movement are unprecedented in recent decades, both in agriculture and with product development, giving rise to the huge upswing of the natural products industry. When enough of us live in a more environmentally friendly way using products made more consciously (with less toxicity and harm to people and nature), we will eventually have healthier bodies and a healthier Earth, which also comes from healthier businesses that don't pollute. When we correct unhealthy lifestyle habits and limit our chemical exposure, we will likely add to our health and vitality, and to our longevity as well.

> **A FEW CLEANING TIPS**
>
> • Safe Home Cleaning Products
>   *(manufactured or homemade)*
>   Vinegar and Baking soda
>   Meyer's Cleaning products
>   Citrasol
>
> • Kitchen Cleanliness
>   Natural soaps
>   Disinfect sponges in microwave
>   or dishwasher
>
> • Plants that help remove toxins from
>   the air:
>   Spider plant,
>   Peace lily,
>   Golden pothos
>
> Many natural products for home and body (such as cosmetics with mostly natural ingredients like coconut oil, and Aloe vera), are available at many stores, and I discuss them in detail in my book *Staying Healthy with Nutrition.*

HYGIENE - OUR PERSONAL ENVIRONMENT

Staying clean, inside and out, is another important health habit. Washing our body is a daily routine that is ideally part of modern living. Exercise and sweating helps clean us from inside out, as we can eliminate toxins. Protecting ourselves from germs with a clean kitchen, awareness of clean food, rotating foods and clearing out old or spoiled items, and learning clean food preparation in our kitchen, are good beginnings.

"Cleaning our food creates a healthy mood for your daily bowlful."

—ARGISLE

Inner cleansing, through juice fasting, or elimination diets (avoiding certain foods and habits) are other useful activities to consider. Giving our bodies a break from foods every so often, and even more importantly, taking breaks from substance use and abuse, is a valuable healing process. I believe a good detox program is important for all of us, as described in my book, The Detox Diet, 3rd Edition (2012).

ACCIDENTS

Although many would consider accidents as "causes" of disease and injury, are they really? How many traumas are really "accidents?" In retrospect, people often realize that they weren't paying attention to more subtle cues or intuitions, or just basic common sense, such as not watching the road when driving because of texting or talking on the phone or even being upset, with your mind racing and making you unaware. When these experiences occur, look at your presence of mind and attention, altered states, or psychoactive substance use to see how they may have played a role. Stress and fatigue can often lead to accidents, and so the accident is in fact a "secondary symptom" telling us about a possible primary symptom. An "accident" often stops us from doing something and changes our direction. Whatever crisis we experience can also be considered an opportunity. (*In Eastern Medicine and language the word for crisis means both danger and opportunity.*) Something positive often comes out of accident experiences, unless of course, there was a premature death, murder, or someone killed by a drunk driver. Whatever happens in life, it is a healthy approach to seek understanding and then make our best efforts to improve the situation, and listen to guidance or learn how to prevent it in the future.

SECONDARY CAUSES:

- **INFLAMMATION**

- **INFECTIONS**

- **IMMUNE DYSFUNCTIONS**

- **METABOLIC DYSFUNCTIONS**

Secondary causes are a result of some of the primary factors. Whether we are balanced or not, even if we have a good diet, exercise regularly, manage our stress, and get quality sleep, at times we can still experience energetic, biochemical, and/or physiological breakdowns or imbalances. Of course, they are less likely to occur with a regular, healthy lifestyle, yet are still possible. A secondary cause means that other factors, such as deficiency and toxicity from our diet and other exposures can lead to problems like an infection or immune imbalance.

INFLAMMATION

Inflammation is a first response the healthy body makes to any irritating physical or emotional factor. It is a key immune response to any foreign or external agent that enters our body, but in excess can lead to numerous symptoms and diseases, from simple aches and pains to diabetes, cardiovascular disease, or heart attacks. But healthy inflammatory responses protect us from infection, tissue damage, and can help build new tissue. It is a healing response when in balance. Excessive inflammation can further worsen immune responses, lead to inflamed tissues, cause pain, and is the basis for many other chronic health problems. Acute exposures to irritants or pathogenic microbes, as well as years of chronic exposure to certain foods, oxidants and toxins, can cause inflammation. A diet high in acidic foods (meats, processed foods with refined sugars and flour, and fried foods) along with environmental and food chemical exposures – also can cause inflammation, stress the body, and damage the immune system. These day-to-day factors may not cause any significant immediate problems, but over time the constant assaults can hurt the body. The beginning process of chronic disease may follow an initial inflammatory response. Also, being obese contributes to inflammation, and losing weight helps quiet the overactive inflammatory response.

Many early signs of deeper health problems begin with inflammatory issues with our organs and blood vessels. These include elevated blood pressure or blood sugar, and high cholesterol, which is a sterol that responds to soothe inflammation. Although many of these early diseases don't usually make us feel ill in the moment, statistically they are predictable for illness if not reduced. That's why it's so important to have regular physical check-ups and blood tests to detect these crucial early risk factors. **This is where Western technology helps us to assess our health or disease potential.**

CHRONIC PERSISTENT INFLAMMATION => DISEASE

Inflammation is the body's first response to any irritant, damage, or foreign organism. If you accidently hit your hand with a hammer, get stung by a bee, burn yourself, or have an infection – the inflammatory response is set in motion. Eating foods that are not compatible with your metabolism or your immune system may also trigger inflammation. And so begins a cascade of cellular and molecular events, resulting in the four cardinal signs of inflammation – redness, swelling, heat, and pain. All of these responses are designed to remove the damage (or irritation) from your body and repair the tissue. It is a normal healing response. Where it becomes damaging, is when inflammation continues beyond its useful cycle and puts stress on other body systems.

In addition to inflammation, other dietary and emotional factors can influence the progression of disease to which Western medicine typically pays minimal attention (although this is changing), such as with cardiovascular disease risk potential. NEW Medicine addresses behaviors to help prevent other costly health problems as well.

For example, in cardiovascular disease, the blood vessels can become damaged or inflamed by tiny tears or irritants. Then the body's attempt to repair these leads to plaque, made up of cholesterol, fibrin, platelets, etc. The inflammation that was originally initiated to heal the blood vessel can cause further plaque. What can damage the vessel at this point are reactive immune cells and chemical oxidants or free radical chemicals, (unstable molecules that can inflame the body) produced by the immune cells.

The wisest approach is to identify risk factors that can contribute to illness, and then aim to prevent the problems, or slow their progress, through education and motivation for change. **Lifestyle factors to focus on first include: diet, exercise, weight loss, stress reduction and psychological support.** By following a nutrient-rich and alkaline diet (lots of greens and veggies) along with specific nutrients (mostly minerals), one can help reduce the inflammatory aspects of any disease. When we have disease risks based on family history, or decades of bad habits, we must be even more diligent in our actions going forward. Even with the ever-present cancer concern and the importance of genetic risk factors, it is well documented that a high percentage of cancers are related to lifestyle—dietary choices, chemical use and exposure, smoking of course, as well as stress and emotions—and our environment, from soil to space.

INFECTIONS AND MICROBES

Many physicians consider infection as a primary disease issue. I believe the body's state of health, i.e. *the body terrain,* has more to do with whether we get sick or not. "Healthy bodies do not get sick, at least very easily." It takes a weakened or congested state for germs to live and multiply and then cause problems.

Often, infections are treated with antibiotics regardless of whether they are caused by a bacteria or a virus. These days more people are aware of this and more doctors are supportive of 'watch and heal' when they suspect the infection is viral. Bacterial infections most often should be treated with antibiotic medications, ranging from the original penicillin and sulfa drugs to the more recently developed broad-spectrum antibiotics. Viral infections, such as a cold or the flu, are not helped by antibiotics, yet a patient may ask for antibiotics or the doctor may suggest them to help prevent and treat any secondary bacterial infections, which do occur, especially with deeper respiratory infections. Antibiotics obviously can be life saving in the face of severe bacterial infections; however, as one of the only choices doctors have to treat infections, antibiotics are frequently overused. Many physicians may not be aware of, nor do they have access to, gentler remedies such as antibacterial herbal or homeopathic options. When a viral infection is diagnosed, we can use some anti-viral medicines, such as Zovirax (acyclovir) or Valtrex (vancyclovir) for herpes infections, and there are more recent anti-flu medicines that work minimally at best. Mostly though, we let things heal naturally with time and care.

Infections result not only from bacteria and viruses, but also from yeast/fungi and parasites. Identifying and treating these specific organisms is just as important even though they require more extensive testing to diagnose them, such as stool testing and antibody levels for various microbes. Often it is harder to find insurance coverage for these more in-depth tests. Especially after being treated with antibiotics, it is more common to have a secondary, yeast-overgrowth infection, which are often ignored and under-treated which then leads to further symptoms and disease.

Acidophilus and "healthy" bacteria are called "probiotics." These provide some balance and support healing, protect us from other intestinal infections, and help to rebalance our gut microbes after antibiotic treatment. The intestines represent our important "inner environment" and what we call the "microbiome." This is vital to healthy immunity, good nourishment and overall function.

It is important to identify and treat specific organisms causing the infection to help improve the healing process. Infection and inflammation are two of the most predominant research areas in modern medicine, as is the aspect of preventing infections through vaccinations. Vaccinations, or immunizations with a non-pathogenic version of a microbe, prod the body to form protective antibodies and immune cells to prevent experiencing the disease from later exposure, or to diminish the severity of a deadly infection when applied and utilized properly.

IMMUNE DYSFUNCTIONS

Imbalanced immunity, be it underactive (hypo) or overactive (hyper), is a common issue leading to a variety of health problems. Immune deficiency or weakness reduces the body's ability to fend off microbes leading to frequent infections not eliminated effectively by the sluggish immune cells. However, the more common problems in the West are due to hyperactive immune functions resulting in allergies or autoimmune illnesses. Allergy symptoms—from simple hay fever (grass, weeds and pollens) to reactions to mold, foods, and animal dander (to name a few)—can range from mild to strong and in extreme cases, even to life-threatening reactions.

Genetics also play a role in the potential for hyperimmune states— allergies, asthma and eczema. If the parent experienced any hyper-immune condition, it increases the risk for their children to develop a similar problem. Yet time, diet and lifestyle may alter the expression of these potentials, as well as reverse the allergies. A personal example of this: I was an "allergic" young person who suffered from a runny, itchy nose and skin rashes for years. I found that juice cleansing and cleaning up my diet in my mid twenties, eliminated my symptoms and they have remained mostly absent, although I am still potentially allergic. I can tell that because of some minimal seasonal reactions, or if I eat too many congesting foods, I will experience a return of moderate allergic symptoms.

METABOLIC DYSFUNCTIONS

Metabolism is the process by which our cells convert one chemical into another more useful product that may provide us with energy or cell building blocks; it's also the process by which our body digests food using calories and nutrients to create energy, warmth and what our body needs to thrive. Thousands of chemical reactions are necessary to turn the food we eat into usable building supplies for growing new cells, building proteins and providing energy to our brain and muscles. The regulation of a healthy metabolism also depends on hormones from our endocrine glands (like the thyroid, pancreas, and adrenals) as well as many different catalyzing enzymes that facilitate all the metabolic steps. Vitamins and minerals also play an essential role. If our organs or nutrients become depleted, our metabolism suffers. Also, when stressed we lose energy and no longer burn calories efficiently to keep us warm and trim.

We often say that people who are slender, no matter what they eat, have a good or fast metabolism. Those of us who gain weight easily and struggle to lose it may have a slow or weaker metabolism. The causes of a sluggish metabolism are many—thyroid imbalance, vitamin or mineral deficiencies, missing or ineffective enzymes, organ burnout, to name a few. And yet, many of these problems are easily remedied with simple lifestyle changes. Health and healthy metabolisms can be restored.

DEFINITION OF METABOLISM:
- The ongoing interrelated series of chemical interactions taking place in living organisms that provide the energy and nutrients needed to sustain life
- The chemical activity involving a particular substance in a living organism

There are many factors that contribute to symptoms, illnesses and diseases. Many of these factors are areas where we have some control, and others are inherent. The end point or outcomes are the problems that many people and their doctors treat. As stated numerous times, it's more effective long term to treat the underlying causes, and adjust treatment as healing continues.

NEW Medicine Principles—Review

- There are many factors that contribute to **Health and Healing**, and many of these depend on us and the choices we make daily.

- With **The Health Continuum** we see that we can often choose whether we only focus on illness or disease and fighting to recover from them, or we embrace and work on enhancing our health and vitality.

- As we begin to appreciate the **Underlying Causes of Disease**, we can observe and understand the basic biochemistry and physiology of how many of the common symptoms and diseases arise, and again look at adjusting our lifestyle so that we can generate better health and lessen symptoms and disease.

- **Cells are at the core of the body's health**, and ideally we focus on avoiding deficiency of needed nutrients, while lowering exposure to toxins, so that our cells function optimally.

- As we see in this chapter and the next one about the 5 Keys to Staying Healthy, our **Nutrition, Exercise, and Stress** are essential building blocks for good health, along with addressing our own and our family's behavior patterns that can lead us to medical problems.

- We see that **Epigenetics may trump Genetics**, therefore our behaviors, including food and nutrient choices, may prevent some of our family's inherent medical issues.

- The primary causes lead to the secondary ones—**Inflammation, Immune Imbalance, Infection, and Metabolic Dysfunction**—and these, in turn, often lead to the many symptoms and disease outcomes.

WHAT'S NEXT?
FROM PRINCIPLES TO PRACTICE

Now, let's go into more detail with the actual lifestyle habits that affect our overall health; I call them **the Five Keys to Staying Healthy**. These are behaviors we have nearly 100% control over and it's very clear to me from my practice experience that embracing these essential aspects of our lifestyle and improving areas like diet and exercise, as well as "managing" stress and nourishing a positive attitude towards ourselves and our world, can make a huge difference in our health - lessening symptoms and complaints, lowering medication needs, and making for a happier more vital life, especially as we age.

THE 5 KEYS TO STAYING HEALTHY

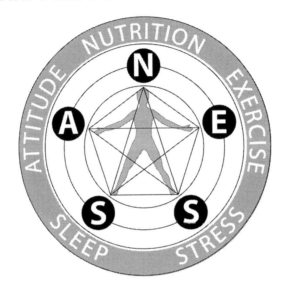

GOOD NUTRITION

REGULAR EXERCISE

STRESS MANAGEMENT

QUALITY SLEEP

HEALTHY ATTITUDES

CHAPTER 3

NEW MEDICINE IN PRACTICE
The Five Keys to Staying Healthy

How we look and feel—our overall health and vitality— are primarily the result of our lifestyle habits, beyond our genetics and family upbringing. It is clear that our health is a result of many factors, most involving the choices we make every day. Of course, there are also choices, over which we have little control, that are made by others and which affect each of us and our environment. The many factors contributing to what we call our *individual lifestyle* include what we eat, our exercise levels, how we manage our stress, our degree of intimacy and personal support, the quality of sleep—all the basic stuff of everyday life. They are all essentially interwoven into the fabric of our existence and of our health. Thus, our wellbeing is primarily up to each of us.

Recent reports suggest that our individual health may be 70% due to choices over which we have control.[1]

Let's review some of the important habits that we may take for granted. These apparently innocuous, unconscious, yet persistent, behaviors contribute greatly to the breakdown or stressing of the body. Some of these could be our daily sugar treats, our one or two cups of coffee to help us through the day, alcoholic drinks to transition from work to home, or our general diet and food choices, especially if we focus on the less healthy ones. What we consume and when, can also affect our sleep, stress, and rest. Just a century ago, people didn't typically live as long as we do today. Even though we have the potential to live long and be vital, we can undermine this privilege by how we live day to day. We see more problems than ever before because of habits like smoking, higher fat diets and refined food choices, and addictions of all kinds, be they drugs or appliances such as computers, televisions and cell phones (and their electromagnetic exposures), and even toxic relationships. Our more sedentary, technology-focused lifestyle actually increases the incidence of many diseases. We see connections between such choices and our health, beginning early in our lives—the dramatic rise in childhood obesity and diabetes are just two of many examples in our current society.

These areas of lifestyle are mostly common health sense and the best way I know to prevent disease. How you engage in these Five Keys makes you tick or sick, and hopefully you would rather be healthy and vital, living to your full potential. Understanding these principles and learning how to apply them will lay the groundwork for building your health and the health of our planet as well. For example, when we use less processed foods and eat more fresh foods, we lessen the amount of packaging, manufacturing and chemical outgassing going into our air and water (as well as our bodies). When we have a less meat-focused diet and less cows grazing our lands, we will produce less methane gas (which contributes to Global Warming) from the steer's excrement. Our whole world, and especially the US, needs to become "more natural" in its focus on health with less chemical use, both personally and in our local environments.

When not feeling at our best, our lifestyle activities are the first area to assess in our health review. To get to know yourself better you might ask:

- What needs healing in my life? My diet, relationships, confidence?
- What changes are needed for healing or rebalancing to occur?
- Am I willing and able to commit to these changes?
- Am I holding back on my health activities? If so, why?

Of course, it is easier to ask such questions than to actually make the changes needed to enhance our wellbeing. Each of these inquiries is complex and meaningful, and each may require deep contemplation, and possibly the guidance of a good counselor. Taking action in these areas empowers us to make a difference for ourselves. Many of us require reprogramming as well as emotional support to make changes in our basic habits. Figuring out how to incorporate these transitions smoothly into our lives is crucial to improving our health, lowering costs and preventing disease.

We can do all the right things and still get sick, so we should not feel like failures when we become ill, but embrace illness as a learning process. Health and medical issues may be mysterious, and it can be challenging to figure out causes and treatments, yet for the most part, when taking good care of ourselves, we attain and maintain better health and vitality and are less susceptible to disease. As with many things in life, ensuring that you have a solid foundation is a good way to proceed.

NUTRITION

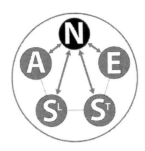

What we ingest (eat, drink, and breathe, even put on our body) is arguably the most important building block of good health, since our cells and tissues only thrive when they are provided with the vital nutrients we need. Simply stated, "Eat as close to Nature as possible and minimize processed and junk foods and chemicals." Of course, there are many other healthy dietary habits, such as eat a balanced diet, chew your food well, relax when eating, and don't eat too much, especially late in the day.

NUTRITIONAL CORNERSTONE FOR GOOD HEALTH

"Eat Wholesome Foods and Avoid Junk and Chemicals"

Most of you know what "junk foods" are and where they fit (or don't) into a healthy diet. Wholesome foods are whole/real foods, especially fresh fruits and vegetables, packaged by Nature (meaning unprocessed), organically and locally grown whenever possible. This also includes grains, nuts, seeds, legumes, fresh eggs, etc. Most processed foods have been heated, treated and refined, and are typically packaged in wasteful plastic; ideally these are only a small part of the diet if they are eaten at all. Avoid foods containing genetically modified organisms foods (often referred to as GMO foods) until we know for sure that they are safe; note that most non-organic corn and soy are genetically modified. There is much to learn about good nutrition and healthy diets, especially when we relate it to each unique individual. What's the right way to eat for each of us? Finding balance is one of the main keys to our lifelong health.

PERSONAL FOOD CHOICES

On occasion, I have taken back items bought by my family and friends, especially those with poor vision who cannot read the small print on the labels. When reading a food label, major concerns are: too much sugar, food colorings like red dye, preservatives, or pork casings on chicken sausages (since I don't eat pork). My personal choice is not to eat four-legged animals, yet I do consume some poultry and fish, and at times eat a vegan diet. I also avoid dairy products such as cow's milk, ice cream and most cheese, although I occasionally consume small amounts in a particular dish, or some feta made from sheep or goat milk in a salad. Even with organic items, I am careful with such things as corn chips and guacamole, gluten-free cookies and Coconut Bliss (dairy-free ice cream that is way too good!). And because I love to eat (mostly good foods), I also need to detoxify regularly and follow a limited menu for periods of time. When eating a balanced diet every day however, I find I need less cleansing and detox.

"Avoid Food-icide." —ARGISLE

Overall, I focus my diet on vegetables and make them the main part of my lunch and dinner, along with some grains and beans, with some fish or poultry or some local organic eggs for protein. Occasionally, we all go overboard at a birthday party or holiday feast, or perhaps with a popcorn movie habit. The ultimate battle is between what's healthy now for each of us, and how our choices add up as an investment—our health portfolio—over time and even our lifetime. So, I adapt my lifestyle to make it better. How do you apply what you know to create a healthy diet for yourself?

Unlocking Your Nutrition Wisdom

- What are your issues and challenges around food?

- Do you live to eat or eat to live?

- What will help you be your best nutritionally?

- What are your food priorities?

- What 7 key foods do you believe best support your overall wellbeing? (Ideally, these are foods that you like and are also healthy for you.)

- How would you rate your daily diet—healthy or full of processed foods?

- Do you use mood and energy altering substances daily, like caffeine, sugar, and alcohol? How often?

- Do your family members eat differently and how does that affect you?

- Do you know how to prepare simple and tasty meals?

- Do you know how to shop for good foods and good deals?

- Are you willing to invest extra money for better foods?

There are many mobile Apps available to help you shop, read labels and find the nutritional content of foods based on the brand name or bar code. These include information on additives, chemicals, GMO[2] content and even country of origin - e.g. Shopwell, Fooducate, Buycott, The Food Ambassador and True Food. More details and reviews can be found at: 50 Best Apps for Food Labels.[3]

DETOXIFICATION & ELIMINATION DIETS

Detoxification is a general term that encompasses simply avoiding certain foods or substances like caffeine or alcohol, to specific cleansing diets and various detoxification programs and supplements. Elimination diets could involve avoiding certain foods for some time, to assess changes and how you feel, or just staying away from SNACC's (an acronym for Sugar, Nicotine, Alcohol, Caffeine, and Chemicals). An occasional elimination diet can benefit nearly everyone, as long as you consume nourishing foods; elimination is often the first step for assessing food allergies, sensitivities, or any food reactions. Ideally, it is both part of general medical care and healthy self-care. The overall message is that we should not be dependent on any food or substance for energy or emotional needs. Thus, we should be able to take a break from coffee, sugar, alcohol, as well as dairy and wheat products—often considered the most overindulged food and substances—to give your body a healthy boost. I truly believe that if our entire nation did this for three weeks, half of people's symptoms and medical conditions would be ameliorated.

"Reduce excesses, but not excessively." —ARGISLE
The converse is also true, *"Moderation in all things, even moderation."*

Once we feel better, we may choose to begin bringing the individual foods back into our diet to see how we feel from a new exposure to them. Ideally we test one food every day or two. I have written extensively on these topics in *The Detox Diet* and *The False Fat Diet*, (which are also integrated in an article called Purification Process on my clinic's website, www.pmcmarin.com.)

Key Nutrition Guidelines

- Eat mostly fresh foods packaged by Nature, not manufactured.

- Focus on vegetables and good quality proteins, plus fresh fruits.

- Know what you're eating and understand food labels (avoid artificial ingredients and toxins).

- Minimize SNACCSs—Sugar, Nicotine, Alcohol, Caffeine, and Chemicals.

- Create a menu plan and eat a balanced diet.

- Eat the right amount of food for you and avoid overeating.

- Eat at the right times for your body and digestion - not too much food at one time nor too late in the day.

- Eat a nourishing breakfast, a good lunch and a lighter dinner.

- Eat in a relaxed setting, without stress or distractions like TV.

- Chew your food well—this is crucial for good digestion.

- Relax a bit after eating for best digestion.

- Learn about food combining and simple eating—not too many different foods at once.

- Learn about the glycemic index of foods—how foods affect your blood sugar.

- Avoid too much restaurant and institutional food, which often contains excessive fats, salt and sugars, and the risk of germs.

- Minimize salt (sodium) intake as well as fried oils and creamy sauces.

- Take time off from indulgences, like a day a week, or a week a month

- Consider periods of detoxification and cleansing.

- Learn about safe food handling and preparation.

- Find out if you are allergic to certain common foods like wheat, dairy, etc.

- Make sure you drink enough clean water daily.

"Peace begins in the kitchens and pantries, gardens and backyards, where our food is grown and prepared. The energies of nature and the infinite universe are absorbed through the foods we eat and are transmuted into our thoughts and actions." [4]   —MISHO KUSHI

EXERCISE

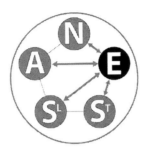

A Consistent and Balanced Exercise Program is Crucial to Good Health. We are designed to move, lift, swing and stretch. Exercise, in its varied forms, stimulates metabolism, circulation, oxygenation, lymphatic activity, and neurological function; strengthens our immune system; reduces stress; lessens inflammation, and with endorphin enhancement, exercise improves our overall attitude. A consistent program of balanced exercise supports the body and helps prevent or improve so many health issues. Depression is one example where regular exercise often helps, by improving mood and energy, reducing anxiety and promoting better sleep.

THE BEST EXERCISE PROGRAM

"Do you know what your best exercise is?" Many will answer, "walking" or "swimming." The BEST exercise program is "**the one that you'll do**." I find that when people are given suggestions that are beyond their ability to enact, they won't do anything. Of course, there are many aspects in regard to healthy exercise to support the body and avoid injury. We could also say this about dietary changes and the individuality of what we choose to eat.

A Balanced Fitness Program includes:

- **Some exercise daily** with a goal of 7-10 hours of physical activity each week.

- **Stretching**—for flexibility, also good before and after aerobics and/or weights.

- **Aerobic activity**—running, hiking, biking, or swimming, for endurance, cardiovascular health and detoxification (sweating).

- **Toning**—using weights or resistance exercises, for strength and muscle mass.

- **Energy balancing**—yoga, qigong, and tai chi (especially helpful for elders).

- **Mood enhancing**—dance and all aerobics support the feel good "endorphins."

Even with physical limitations, do what you can, from isometrics to using a stretch band, or even stretching or yoga in a chair. You can also do deep breathing along with tightening and relaxing muscles while sitting or working at your computer. Remember, if you aren't already exercising regularly, have a physical exam before you begin and build your endurance at a healthy pace.

My attitude is (and it could be yours, too): "This is the only body I have and I am going to treat it with love." Once we develop this approach, giving our body some vitamin L (Love), we develop an internal commitment to being healthy. With this essential feeling of body respect and love, we will often tend to eat better, exercise more regularly, learn to manage stress more effectively and take better overall care of ourselves.

Evaluate Your Exercise Program

- Do you enjoy exercise?

- Which activities do you like most?

- Do you exercise daily? If not, how often?

- How many hours of exercise do you average weekly?

- Do you dislike exercise and find it hard to pick something that motivates you?

- Do you stretch daily?

- Do you run or engage in other active aerobic activity?

- Do you lift weights or do other strength and muscle development activities?

- Do you like to go to a gym, or do you prefer to be on your own?

- Do you like team activities?

- Have you been accused of being an exercise fanatic or exercising too much.

- Have you injured yourself from any of your exercise activities?

- Do you sense that exercise is helpful for your long-term health?

- What can you do to improve or enhance your overall fitness program?

STRESS

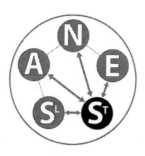

The topic of stress is so instrumental to our overall health, while its impact on our health is not sufficiently understood. Since there are many related levels and factors, this section is a bit longer than the other 5 Keys. Stress is a term that suggests that the increased demands placed on ourselves to deal with day-to-day life are above and beyond those we are able to handle successfully. This has to do with the way we react and respond to our life experiences. What triggers stress is unique to each person. For some it might be a challenging relationship at home or work, bills to pay, or watching the many varied worldwide catastrophes on the news. It might be something severe such as losing a loved one, or being abused by someone, or something as simple as our children or spouse leaving their dirty dishes or clothes around the house. We are also affected by climate changes and the barometric pressure. Overall, stress is an "adaptation response," or as Hans Selye[5] originally defined it in 1936, *"Stress is the non-specific response of the body to any demand for change."*[6] He measured this in terms of physiological activities of the autonomic nervous system that oversees our body's activities. Since Selye's time, it has been established that the mind and our perceptions play a key role in what is stressful to each of us.

No one definition of stress has been universally accepted. Some include the acute reaction to external events such as war or environmental assaults. Others include cellular stress responses such as to infectious agents, and even exercise. **Currently, the most broadly accepted concept of stress is the perception that one doesn't have the resources to handle a given situation,** or a feeling of being overwhelmed with what one has to handle.[7]

HEALTHY STRESS AND CHRONIC STRESS

There is also "healthy stress." This includes a desire to do well on a test or interview, having a response to actual danger (not just the fear of a possible future danger), such as being threatened by someone or running from a wild animal. With healthy stresses, we have an appropriate physiological (adrenal gland and adrenaline hormone) response to provide us the energy, mental capacity and ability to react quickly and respond wisely. This kind of response typically subsides once the danger passes. The main concern for our health is chronic stress, which is the persistent worry and fear about things that might happen, or reliving past events.

> There are many types and sources of stress, especially in our modern times and busy lives. These can all lead to inflammation and body tensions, even if it is problems with a loved one, our local community, or the world. These varied stresses include:
>
> - **Physical stress** from intense exercise or competitive events as well as injury or illness, such as flu or bronchitis or any long-term illness or surgery, pregnancy or travel.
>
> - **Emotional stress** from relationships, love (or the lack of it), marriage and divorce, raising children, taking care of a sick loved one, anger, jealousy, fears and phobias such as worrying about germs, and standing up for ourselves.

- **Mental stress** from the demands of our work (or school), deadlines, taking tests, speaking in public, or just too many decisions to make.

- **Financial stress** from money concerns and paying bills, the stock market, rising mortgage payments, how your partner is spending the family finances, or how the government is spending our money.

- **Biochemical (oxidative), Pollution, and Electromagnetic stresses** at the level of our cells and tissues from toxins and free radicals or EMF exposures, whether we are aware of it or not, such as with the Fukishima catastrophe.

- **Spiritual and Life stress** from making important life decisions about our future, such as where we'll live or work (job or house hunting, moving), who to be with on a personal level, or what our life's purpose is. Life transitions such as adolescence, pregnancy or aging may also fit into this category.

These various factors do not operate in isolation and in fact often compound one another to intensify our stress response. Having too many stressors without a healthy outlet for relief is a major concern. Music can touch us and calm our soul, as can dancing and going to parties or hanging out with friends and family. Keep in mind that love and personal connection are vital to a healthy you.

What challenges us is uniquely personal. Almost any situation or experience can create a stress response, so the list is endless. It is our point of view that often makes any situation stressful. Lifestyle and general counseling can help us shift our attitudes and this involves getting to know our selves more intimately and honestly. Meditation can help us too. Ideally, an important part of a doctor's practice is helping people and patients handle and learn to adapt to, stressful life situations. The key point is that we learn to recognize and manage our stress, and avoid it whenever possible; this will benefit our overall health.

"Less struggle, more snuggle." —ARGISLE

STRESS AND BODY SYSTEMS

Our Immune Health, Nervous System, Heart, and Digestive Tract appear to be the most sensitive to emotional upset and stress. Chronic stress also affects the muscles, often causing tightness and pain. We get wired and tired and get sick more easily when we exhaust ourselves with worry and struggle. It helps to find daily balances for our anxieties and concerns. What will work for you. Is it regular exercise, in the gym or water therapy like swimming; walking in Nature; or yoga and working with your breath? These all may be helpful to calm the body and nerves. Most of us need less "to-do" and more "to-be" time.

"Take a Health Holiday! Stress less, take a rest, and be blessed."

—ARGISLE

STRESS AND RELATIONSHIPS

Along with work and finances, relationships are often a primary stressor. It is important that we each know how to *handle and respond to the demands and emotions we experience* and that we also learn how to access feelings and express them in positive ways to our loved ones, co-workers, friends and our selves. This begins with making statements that do not blame or attack another, but rather state more clearly how something affects us, how we feel, and how we wish to be acknowledged or treated. One example is a husband or child who doesn't clean up after himself and/or leaves a mess in the kitchen or dishes around the house. You could easily say, "You stupid jerk! Why are you such a slob? If you don't do X, then I am going to do Y." That person may feel attacked and may either retreat hurtfully, or be defensive with a snide comment and begin an outright fight. Another approach would be to say, "I am feeling the stress of caring for this household. I am asking you to help me please by putting your dishes in the sink and doing the dishes a few times a week. I will greatly appreciate that. Thank you." That has more likelihood of getting a positive response and action. When feeling attacked, it's natural to react defensively and protect our selves, or run and hide as in the "fight or flight" response. Any retaliation usually snowballs and soon we have a shouting match, or all out war. When we expect some resistance or a possible fight about some topic, my policy is often to begin by asking or stating, "I would really like your support in this situation." This engages the other person and the innate need to be helpful, appreciated and loved.

One important thing to develop (and I have shared this over the years with patients and the working staff at our medical center) is **"Learn the difference between a reaction and a response."** A *reaction* is a defense response—often instinctual—whereby we attempt to protect our self, our emotions and point of view. Often in this state we have not really heard or received what the other has expressed. Plus, we may feel we are made to look wrong and may attack another. A *response* suggests that we actually took in the communications of the other person, processed them, and responded with some thoughts and feelings; thus, we managed our behavior with some intelligence and care. Aspects involve taking turns speaking and fully listening, and then acknowledging what you heard before responding. Then there is less defensiveness and trying to talk over the other person.

"Beyond compromise is cooperation." —ARGISLE

This whole process is so crucial to healthy relationships, long-term marriages, and really all communications. Of course, our ability to manage stress also depends upon the choices we have made regarding personal and business relationships—the people with whom we have chosen to devote our lives, and the level to which each of these relationships can grow with conscious nourishment. The wiser and clearer we are in our choices, the smoother the relationship ride we will experience, and the more enjoyable and loving it will be for all involved. And when we have not chosen wisely, admit it and move forward as best you can.

FAIR FIGHTING

The Art and Technique of Peacefully "Not" Getting Along!
Fighting can cause pain and often comes from reaction and defensiveness; listening and responding from a level of understanding helps to keep love alive. We can still disagree with our loved ones or co-workers, yet it doesn't mean we have to battle with them. It's better to learn and incorporate methods and develop some level of emotional command to encourage better understanding and healing. "Fair fighting" is a technique I mention to my patients when they struggle with a spouse, for example. This also relates to a

process called the Socratic Dialogue as described in *The Dialogue Game* by Peter Winchell. Fair fighting can help us resolve important differences or accept how they are.

Some Guidelines for Fair Fighting:

- Embrace personal respect and care for one another; this is mutuality/equanimity.

- Take turns and let each other speak without interruption and listen while they are talking, not rehearsing what you are going to say next. You can use a "talking stick"—whoever holds it gets to speak; when they are done, they pass it on.

- Set time limits for each person's turn or the total dialogue.

- When it's your turn, acknowledge what you heard the other say.

- State how you think and feel—not the "blame game" making the other wrong.

- No name calling, threats or ultimatums, yet create clear boundaries.

- Compassion is a key for the goals of understanding and mutual support; put yourself in the other person's shoes.

- Look toward healing solutions and realize that there are always two sides (at least) to any argument, and the solution lies in the cooperation (some say compromise yet that suggests giving up rather than giving something) between the people involved.

- Dare to share your care, even when not in agreement.

- Avoid trying to resolve things when under the influence of alcohol or other substances; anger and reactivity are more predominant with alcohol.

PERSONAL STRESS

Personal communications and relationships are just one example of stress. The demands we place on ourselves are likely the biggest stresses in how we respond to life, not just the actual events. People relate through different levels of stress depending on how sensitive they are, or what their past experiences have been. When something re-stimulates an old wound, it can be quite traumatic, yet to another person, it may not seem like such a big deal.

WHAT ABOUT COUNSELING?

Reviewing your issues with a therapist experienced in listening and reflecting back to you can help you begin to process and heal. Venting sessions can get out some feelings. Also, couples' sessions can be extremely useful at working through conflicts. Managing "reaction vs. response" is a key to reducing chronic stress in our lives, and this is one of the major keys to preventive health. Of course, this doesn't mean we should give up our instincts and abilities to "react" appropriately should we need to.

SOME STRESS REDUCTION TIPS

- **Nutrition**—Avoid too many stimulants like caffeine and excessive sugar. Focus on high-nutrient natural foods to keep the body nourished and relaxed. Chemicals may create increased toxicity and inflammatory stress.

- **Supplements and Herbs**—as needed, support the body and its organs: e.g. for the adrenals use vitamins B and C; plus benefit from herbs like licorice root, ashwaganda, and Siberian ginseng; or support for liver through body detoxification (giving the liver a little rest) along with various nutritional products, such as alpha-lipoic acid or milk thistle herb containing silymarin.

- **Exercise**—Regular physical activity offers a great program for stress reduction. There are also many valued "internal exercises" as tai chi and qigong.

- **Social support**—with a listening, caring friend or family member; with more significant issues, a licensed therapist or counselor would be helpful.

- **Meditation**—deep breathing aids relaxation and stress reduction; programs/methods such as Mindfulness Based Stress Reduction (MBSR) developed by Jon Kabat-Zinn or Heartmath's coherent breathing techniques.[8]

- **Behavior Modification**—learning how to replace undesirable behaviors with more desirable ones through positive or negative reinforcement.

- **Practice Rethinking**—seeing a challenging situation differently and visualize the desired outcome.

- **Attitude**—How do you look at life? Make positive changes to support your mood and energy level.

- **Prayer**—as with meditation, tune into what's right and best for all; as your belief in any higher power. The main prayer might be, "Thy will be done through me."

- **Laugh**—watch a funny movie or TV show.

- **Connect with Nature**—take a short walk – fresh air, trees and water can help us calm down and rebalance.

Stress Self-Inquiry

What causes you stress? There are many possibilities. Learning to know your self and finding ways to cope are keys to managing the common stresses of everyday life.

Take time for self-evaluation.

- What are the most stressful issues or situations I have now?
- Is there a repeating pattern?
- What can I do to lessen the stress? Do I know how?
- What specific stress reduction techniques do I already know?
- How can I manage a stressful situation when I can't change it?
- Do I have the support I need when challenges arise?
- Who are my trusted friends that I can talk with.
- How aware are they of me and my patterns?
- Do I know how to respond rather than react?
- Do I leave or confront?
- Do I run away from intimate interactions?
- Can I handle the truth?
- Do I need more quiet, relaxation and sleep?
- Do I know how to be at peace?

"Tit for tat, my this, your that."
"Let's play each other's part in clear and healing communication."
"No one to blame, no shame to tame; you're the winner in your life's game."

—ARGISLE

SLEEP

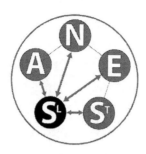

WHAT IS SLEEP?

For humans and most animals, sleep is a period of rest and recharging from the activities and stresses of our daily lives. Sleep is a time for the brain and nervous system to replenish its reserves and to rest our digestive tract, our spine and our muscles. We each have our own sleep patterns and needs. Sleep is a time when we restore our vital functioning and allow our conscious mind to rest and release our subconscious mind to be active. Sleep also changes as we grow and age.

Chronic sleep deprivation has many health consequences including increased risk for infections, heart disease, depression, impaired cognitive functions and more accidents.[9] Fatigue and low motivation also occur frequently when we don't properly recharge our 'batteries.'

Sleep apnea is a common sleep disorder caused by interrupted, or insufficient, breathing and poor oxygenation; this can be related to anatomical interference, weight, allergies, and more. It is more frequently diagnosed now due to increased awareness of the problem, plus easier access to sleep centers, which test and monitor sleep with an overnight sleep study. Snoring can be another aspect of apnea.

HOW MUCH SLEEP DO WE NEED?

Our individual requirement for sleep depends on both the quantity (hours) as well as the quality of our sleep. This involves how deeply we sleep and whether we feel replenished or exhausted when we wake up. We need to go into the slower *theta* waves where we dream in order to become completely recharged. Many of us are partly or fully "sleep deprived." Insomnia is one of the most common complaints seen by physicians, as is fatigue, which is partly due to poor sleep. Some reports have suggested that 50-70 million adults, more than 35% of Americans are sleep deprived.[10] Are you?

WHY DON'T WE SLEEP WELL?

Many of us don't sleep well because we stay up late with TV and computers on, receiving too much light and electricity to support nighttime quiet. Then, often we must awaken earlier than our own rhythm might want us to, using alarms from a clock or cell phone. This is common with jobs and school, and especially challenging for teenagers, who seem to gravitate too late to bed and ever later to arise. If we ingest too many stimulants in our diets (coffee, sugars, chocolate) throughout the day, our sleep often suffers. Having too many stresses and worries diminishes quality sleep. Too much electromagnetic activity (TVs, digital clocks, microwaves, and wifi) in our homes and bedrooms could alter sleep quality. Do you get quality sleep with a partner, or do you sleep better alone? Often, long time couples end up sleeping in different rooms because one snores or they like different covers and room temperatures, or generally have different sleep patterns.

Quality sleep is essential for maintaining good health and includes being able to fall asleep easily and stay asleep; awaken naturally at the right time; and feeling rested and ready for the day. This is important for a healthy, energetic body that can live to its potential.

Assess the Quality your own Sleep

- How often are you satisfied with your current sleep? Daily, weekly, never?

- Do you know your natural sleep needs and sleep cycles?

- How much sleep do you need before you feel rested.

- Do you fall asleep easily and stay asleep through the night?

- Do you wake up during the night?
  - How often?
  - Why?
  - Is it to urinate?
  - Is it anxiety?

- Can you go back to sleep easily if you awaken during the night.

- Do you have nightmares or anxiety-generating dreams? How often?

- Is there a specific cause of poor sleep, like allergies, medications or anxiety?

- Is a change in your sleep patterns?

- Is this change related to life cycles, like menopause or aging?

- What is your state of mind when you wake up?

- Do you feel rested when you wake up?

- Do you need an alarm clock and reset it two or three times before getting up?

- Do you have energy throughout the day, or do you need many jolts of caffeine and sugar, and then alcohol later to relax?

- If you have a sleep partner, how does he, or she, affect your sleep?

There are many consequences of poor sleep—including immune deficiency and subsequent illness, mood and cognitive issues and a general lack of energy and motivation? Sleep experts talk about 'sleep hygiene' as a primary approach to help improve the quality of sleep. In fact, the *New England Journal of Medicine*[11] and the *National Sleep Foundation*[12] recommend behavior change an. 'sleep hygiene' as the primary way to deal with sleep problems, not resorting to pharmaceuticals at first.

Ways to Improve Your Sleep

Before Bed—Sleep Prep

- Be quiet about an hour before bedtime, dim the lights, and turn off computers and TV. Listen to calming music or meditate. Many read something to relax and get sleepy.

- Avoid alcohol, coffee or chocolate, vigorous exercise, or eating too much in the hours before bed.

- Get some fresh air and light exercise if you find that helps you relax. A walk outdoors to see some stars and experience the quiet of night can be helpful.

In the Bedroom

- Make your bedroom a comforting environment that gives you a sense of peace and relaxation.

- Keep your room dark and find the right temperature that helps you sleep—cooler is usually better.

- Make sure your bed and bedroom are used primarily for sleep (or physical intimacy) and not for working on computers or watching television. In general, keep your electromagnetic exposure as low as possible in the bedroom.

If these suggestions don't work, try natural remedies before going on to stronger pharmaceutical medicines, but if you do use medications, do so only as a temporary measure.

EXPLORE THESE NATURAL APPROACHES FIRST

- Melatonin (1-3 mg) taken 30 minutes before sleep (helps align diurnal sleep rhythm but not for people with autoimmune conditions).

- Serotonin supporters like L-tryptophan (500-1500 mg) and 5-HTP (50-200 mg) help with deeper sleep.

- GABA (250-1,000 mg) is a brain and nervous system calmer, and L-theanine (200-400 mg) may support better relaxation of mind and body and help with sleep; these two items are often contained together in products like *Liposomal Zen Liquid* (by Allergy Research Group).

- Calcium Magnesium combinations in equal amounts of 250-500 mg each often helps with relaxation and sleep.

- Herbs like valerian, chamomile (caution for people with allergies to ragweed) and catnip, or formulas like Sleepytime or Nighty Night teas.

Your doctor may prescribe sleeping pills like Ambien or Sonata or more tranquilizer medicines like Ativan or Xanax. These can help break poor sleep cycles with a good sleep, yet all of these are addictive and some can contribute to amnesia or sleep walking.

Overall, try to align with natural sleep as much as possible by lowering your stimulants, improving your exercise, eating well, and lowering electronic exposures later in the day.

Clearly, many health and life situations can affect sleep, such as menopause, getting up frequently to urinate, and/or stress/anxiety conditions, especially as we age. Usually, children sleep quite well and longer than adults, so if they have trouble sleeping, it can be more of a concern. Though teens have a slightly altered sleep cycle compared to adults, their reluctance to wake too early for school is usually biologically based.[13] They need more sleep than adults. Ideally, school should start later for all our young people. For poor sleep, you want to identify the underlying causes. Allergies can be one, as can emotional upset and mental worries. (Sleep issues, specifically Insomnia, are discussed in more detail in my upcoming book *NEW Medicine Solutions*.)

MY SLEEP STORY

It's a challenge for me to sleep very long. I began to have some sleep issues during medical school and internship when I was on call every third or fourth night and often didn't have time to sleep. Then, when I began to cleanse and heal my body in my twenties, I seemed to need less sleep and that aligned with liking to get up early and being ambitious to write books, run a medical practice and have a family.

As we age, many of us tend to need less sleep or have trouble sleeping - not dozing off easily into deep dreams or waking up during the night and being mentally or energetically restless. I sometimes experience the latter. In recent years, I often sleep about a five-hour stretch, awaken, get up and pee, and then relax in bed and either read or do puzzles, meditate or take some relaxing natural product. (Aromatherapy, like lavender, may help some people sleep; mugwort is also known to help sleep and dreams.)

For going to sleep, I have successfully used the natural approaches outlined above: I take 5-HTP or L-Tryptophan, or a combo supplement that contains 3mg melatonin, 200mg GABA, and 300mg Tryptophan. If I wake up during the night, I may take a Zen capsule and a few pumps of the liquid liposomal Zen (both contain L-theanine and GABA). On occasion, or when traveling, I may take a low dose (.25mg) of Xanax (alprazolam) with some Tryptophan, and then I read for a bit and go back to sleep for 2-3 hours and often dream. I only do this if I am up before 4 am or haven't slept at least five hours so I don't sleep too late and interfere with my day.

That's how I balance my sleep patterns. Of course, if I've eaten too late, or have increased stresses, sleep may be more challenging. Luckily, I don't use caffeine or stimulants and have a good attitude, and I have learned how to release worries, or write things down that are on my mind before going to bed. All these practices may help.

ATTITUDE

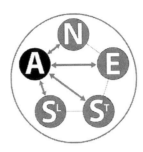

Thousands of studies correlate mental activities and attitudes with health behaviors and disease outcomes. What happens upstairs in our mind, with our thoughts, affects the body and how it functions; this in turn, affects our mind and mental capacities. Since everything we do and consume leads to what makes up our current body–brain–mind, each change we make has the capability of altering our whole being positively or negatively. Relaxing both our mind and body, helps us to reduce our stress and ease our muscle tension and tightness. Exercise, massage, and meditation are three strategies to support relaxation and stress management. Our Mind-Body Balance affects all the other factors of our lives. And this starts with our attitude towards life and self. These attitudes mostly come from our life experiences—how our parents act, think and express themselves; our upbringing; our relationships, and more.

"As Above, so Below." —HERMES TRISMEGISTUS

What I have learned and believe: "Our mind affects our body, and our body affects our mind. What goes on in the cosmos affects life on Earth."

Attitude is the fifth Key to Staying Healthy, but it could easily be the first. Our attitudes influence our lifestyle choices and those choices affect our health directly. Our beliefs about life and what we tell ourselves in the privacy of our own mind—our "self talk"—can be optimistic or pessimistic. When you examine your own attitudes, are they positive and encouraging, or negative and undermining. For instance, compare these differences in attitude:

- "I can improve my health and heal, or I will always be ill."

- "I can make the changes that I know are best for my body and health, or why bother making any changes, what's the point? They won't make a difference."

- "I love myself and feel blessed with my life, or I don't like the person I am and the life I am living, I don't like the way my life is unfolding."

- "I can accomplish my goals, or I can't."

Martin Seligman, PhD[14] introduced the ideas of learned helplessness and learned optimism to the field of positive psychology. He has shown that optimism can be learned even if we start off helpless or hopeless. His work developed into the very practical cognitive behavioral therapy. This teaches us how to view issues differently. His popular book summarizing this work is *Learned Optimism: How to Change Your Mind and Your Life.*[15]

"Well-being cannot exist just in your own head. Well-being is a combination of feeling good as well as actually having meaning, good relationships and accomplishment." —MARTIN SELIGMAN

Healthy attitudes underlie all lifestyle habits. When I changed my diet back in 1975 and started to feel better, I began to make statements like, *"it matters what I put into my mouth; everything I eat becomes part of me. I love my body and thus I want to do what's best for me."*

This approach sets in motion a whole cascade of positive effects. When loving myself, I want to be nurturing and not mistreat myself with poor food choices, substance abuse, or negative thoughts as some examples. So many poor lifestyle habits come from the feelings people have about their self worth, as well as old mental patterns about who we are, which come from parents, siblings or others we encounter in life. I see this with people who abuse themselves with drugs, foods and other substances, when they perceive themselves as victims, less worthy and less deserving. **Our habits reinforce our belief system about what we expect and deserve in life.**

I realize that shifting attitudes and behaviors is not easy; it may mean challenging and changing some of our core beliefs and habits that we have built over decades. Research shows that if the mind doesn't change first, then changes in behavior typically don't last.

"If one cannot change a situation that causes his suffering, he can still choose his attitude. We who lived in concentration camps can remember the men who walked through the huts comforting others, giving away their last piece of bread. They may have been few in number, but they offer sufficient proof that everything can be taken from a man but one thing: the last of human freedoms—to choose one's attitude in any given set of circumstances, to choose one's own way." —VICTOR FRANKL

In some ways, this is the most important aspect of a healthy lifestyle—to shift and support our belief that we are creating a healthy body-mind and a fulfilling life by treasuring each breath deeply within ourselves. In searching for optimal wellness, it's best to seek out people, practitioners and friends who will support our healthy attitudes and who can help us change our unhealthy ones. The mind—the passionate, stressed, and uncontrolled mind—can generate havoc in people's lives. Learning to relax and be 'quiet' can create moments of peace, which our body–mind appreciates. However, we may only pay special attention to this when we are ill or when we are experiencing psychological imbalances.

"The mind is probably the most underutilized health resource we have. Our thoughts, beliefs, attitudes and practices can set the stage for a resilient, resourceful response to stress or illness, or a collapse into fear and helplessness. What we know now is that not only can we become aware of the thought patterns that help or hinder us, we can also change them with practice and persistence. And when we change our thinking patterns, our brain also changes to make it easier to think that way in the future." —MARTY ROSSMAN, MD

Learning and practicing mental and physical relaxation exercises, like meditation (or yoga, qigong or tai chi), can make a difference. Since most medical issues and healing are affected by stress and psycho-emotional conflicts—in the past we referred to them as "psychosomatic" problems—they can be improved with a peaceful (non-reactive) mind and relaxing from stress. Medical specialists often have a name for such psychosomatic problems in their area of expertise, such as Irritable Bowel Syndrome for GI doctors or tension headaches, anxiety and insomnia for family doctors.

Visualizing the body or a specific part in its healed state may help in the healing process. This requires that we calm ourselves first, especially the mind and emotions, which allows imagery and healing to happen. I often have told people, *"Get out of the way and healing will happen."*

EXAMPLE OF A CALMING EXERCISE FOR ENERGY FLOW

One of my favorite internal exercises is a breathing pattern described in a book I read long ago entitled, *The Secret of the Golden Flower*, by R. Wilhelm with an introduction by Dr. Carl Jung.[16] Here's my adapted version.

Lying on your back, place one hand over your lower belly and the other on your heart area (can also be done with the arms at your sides). With eyes closed, breathe slowly and deeply into your lower abdomen, letting the breath move up to your upper chest as your body begins to relax.

Visualize a ball of white or golden light below your feet. Feel a wave of energy like an ocean wave begin at your feet and rise up and over the front of your body as you breathe in, and then feel the wave of energy go down your back as you breathe out.

This creates a circle of energy moving up the front and down the back, in a similar way to the energy flow through the acupuncture meridians or your chakras. I like the feeling of an ocean wave washing over me or light cleansing me and bringing healing energy in, and letting go of pain, fear, worries, or whatever is troubling me. I believe this helps the body feel lighter and clearer and removes some of the blocks that lead to pain and disease.

Simply stated, illness is dis-ease, or lack of ease with self and life. Illness is also resistance to change while healing represents growth and awareness, learning and evolution. When resistances get out of the way, energy flows and we begin to heal, which is to come into a new balance. Aaah! This idea of energy flow is an important part of Chinese Medicine and Acupuncture. Of course, illness is not all in the mind, yet when we ease up and learn to relax and reduce our stress, many health issues improve, or don't begin at all.

"Lax is not the same as relax." —ARGISLE

Some ideas to help shift your attitude from "glass half-empty" to "glass half-full."

- Seek out friends or practitioners who will support your healthy attitudes and who can help you change your unhealthy ones.

- Exercise your motivation muscles. Set a goal for yourself that you can commit to and complete, such as "This week I am going to walk for 30 minutes every other day.. When you keep that commitment and see that you can, your attitude will shift to believing in yourself more and being more positive.

- Learn and practice meditation, yoga, qigong or tai chi, to make a difference.

- Contribute to someone else's healing through your support. Give of yourself by helping other less fortunate and you get more back.

- Visualize the whole body, or a specific part, in its healed state to help in the healing process. This requires that we calm our mind and emotions first so that healing imagery can take effect.

MIND—BODY—LIFE CONNECTIONS

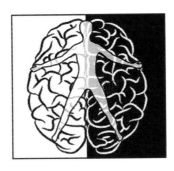

There are several other areas to tune into for a healthy vital life aligned with who we are most deeply. We all want be as aware as we can to cultivate the best life we can with love, prosperity and health. There are many subtle levels to our beings, and as with diet, we can do well or not pay too close attention. Check out these next few topics that embrace the many aspects of human life focusing on underlying causes of health challenges. These deeper levels include:

- **KNOW YOUR CYCLES and RHYTHMS**

- **INNER GUIDANCE**

- **DISCOVER YOUR GIFTS and PURPOSE**

METAPHYSICIANS

During the 1980s and 90s, I was part of and eventually president of a group of MDs and DOs called *Metaphysicians*, who believed that there was an important factor missing in modern medicine—namely that spirituality was essential in healthcare practice. People are much more than a physical body that can break or break down and needs to be fixed. Yes, we are material beings, yet feelings, thoughts, and spirits as well. Sometimes it's our mind or spiritual clarity that needs fixing or realignment. The monthly meetings were rich in presentations and conversations. I miss that group of like-minded docs, and the experience we shared has added value to my understanding and work.

While the discussions that follow fall outside the conventional Western Medical approach, I believe they are an essential part of staying truly healthy.

KNOW YOUR CYCLES & RHYTHMS

Knowing your natural rhythms and staying connected to Nature's Seasonal Cycles are vital keys to Staying Healthy and this can be at all levels—Physical, Mental, Emotional and Spiritual.

I appreciate and sense the connection between the cycles of nature and our mind/body wellbeing. Bethany Argisle, my associate and ally, coined the term "Cycle-ologist" for someone interested in this subject. What this means is being aware of how our needs vary with the changes in seasons and climates, as well as over the seasons of our lifetime. For instance, in the colder, wintery months we need to find ways to keep warm and eat heartier and heating foods. In the spring, doing some detox and cleansing prepares us for eating lighter and staying cool and hydrated during the warmer summer months. I suggest that you journal your cycles and life experiences. This awareness also assists in seeing others more clearly and how our cycles may be aligned with theirs.

These various cycles have to do with more than just food and seasonal eating. They have to do with our physical, mental and emotional energies as well as our creativity. Don't you sense that at times you have more creative spark, or stronger physical energy, or the ability to handle emotions?

LIFE CYCLE EXAMPLE

From my early studies of Chinese texts, I embrace the idea of three major cycles of life, each lasting about 29 years. The first cycle is "getting to know our self" where we learn who we are, our likes and dislikes, our strengths and weaknesses. Then around the ages of 27-29 we experience the first major "doyo," or "life change," period. In Western astrology, this is known as the "Saturn Return" as it takes this planet 29.7 years to complete one orbit around the sun. At this first transition, we move into our "life path" or "career" cycle with a focus on "what do we do with who we are," why are we here, what we have to share with the world, and how does it support us in return, as a livelihood. Then, in our later 50s (56-59), we transition into our third cycle, the "spiritual" or "destiny" years, when we are ideally doing things that truly fulfill us and feed us spiritually. Thus, it helps to know our selves well and to be attuned to the focus of these three primary cycles to make the most out of our life. These cycles play out in many people's lives along with the challenges that can arise during the transition periods.

"Adjusting to change is a benefit (and resource) of a healthy being."
—ARGISLE

We each have our own cycles/biorhythms that relate to physical, mental and emotional energies, and these are accessible to us, although usually less obvious than the female menstrual cycle. It's vital to our health and consistent well being to be aware of, and adaptable to, these many levels of personal and planetary cycles. This topic is so important (and underappreciated) that my first book *Staying Healthy with the Seasons* was dedicated to it. Cycle awareness can begin simply with the basic "Back-to-Nature" message of eating wholesome natural seasonably based foods, and then extend to our own personal rhythms and further to the great cycles of the cosmos. I believe this is essential for maintaining our good health.

INNER GUIDANCE

We can learn a great deal about ourselves on this journey toward better health. **One key discovery is that our inner guidance already has many of the answers we need, IF we can tune in to it.** Perhaps another way to say this is that our most precious knowledge may lie in our subconscious mind and in our cells. When we trust our Self—when we listen and allow ourselves to be moved by our inner voice and intuition—many health problems and accidents may be prevented. Commonsense about health and habits goes a long way, and our inner Self has a lot of commonsense! *Trust your rhythm and your gut instincts, and persevere to achieve what you believe.*

Often, our keys to healing, especially with more challenging health problems, have to do with listening more deeply. An integrative medicine approach allows us to get deeper into the causes and factors contributing to any dis-ease. This process of discovery is almost always a personal one. As we begin with the belief that the deeper levels of our body/mind, our inner psyche and subconscious know what is out of balance and helps us see what is needed for healing to occur, we can restore our natural balance and homeostasis.

One way to begin using inner guidance is by asking different questions of our self than are typically asked by most people and their doctors. Often, people simply want to know what's wrong, and they will tell their doctor when and where they are hurting, *"Please, fix me or make this go away. Give me something I can take to get rid of this pain, allergy, headache, or indigestion."* As we have previously discussed, this approach generally leads to "symptom fixing," not to true long-term healing.

> Bernie Siegel, MD shared his knowledge and experience with patients who expressed themselves with journal keeping and drawing from their inner vision in his early books, *Love, Medicine, and Healing,*[17] *Peace, Love, and Healing* and many more.[18] As a cancer surgeon, he worked with people with serious illness, and shaved his head to better connect with his bald patients.

Exploring Healing By Interviewing Your Body & Symptoms

Here are some questions that might help you learn to listen to your inner guidance and lead you to a healing path. Pick those that feel most appropriate for you to ask your inner self, your intuition, or your dreams. Do this before bed and write the down those you've chosen on paper, or in your journal.

- Body, what is going on inside me now?
- What are you trying to tell me, dear body?
- How well do I sense that I am listening to my body's messages and choices?
- What is my current health challenge?
- Why do I have this problem now?
- What was/is out of balance that has allowed my body to become ill?
- What conflicts or issues are involved in my problem?
- What mental, spiritual or other non-physical factors may be involved in my symptoms?
- What is needed for healing to occur?

- Where does healing need to occur?

- Is there anything I need to let go of, or to add?

- Is there a symbol, or story, for this illness, symptom, or the healing process?

- What opportunity does this health challenge provide for me to make changes in my life?

- Given what I now know about my symptoms, do I have a new and better plan for healing, and if so what is it?

- When do I feel my best, and what contributes to that?

I encourage you to interview your own body in this way, listen to and track your cycles, and see what you learn. Pay attention over the years to see if your health is impacted at certain times or seasons. Keep a personal journal to record your thoughts and feelings, your dreams (both nighttime and daytime dreams), aspirations and life activities. Whatever you are inclined to record is what's right for you.

"Through journaling and daily reading and writing, we can form new healthy habits."
— ARGISLE

Question yourself before you go to sleep or when you first wake up, and then listen deeply and openly to what comes to mind. Write your questions down before you go to sleep and ask that your dreams reveal to you the clear message—an answer to conflict, decisions or guidance needed. If you meditate, you can also write your

"GOOGLE YOUR BODY"

Ask deeply within and listen for the answers to arise in your psyche. We can do this with a meditation exercise or ask questions before you go to sleep. (I recommend that people write them down). Ask your dreams to reveal the answers to you. This is based on the belief that our body/brain functions as a bio-computer and knows all of what we need to know.

questions down beforehand and allow your body, heart, mind and spirit to review them and delve within to reveal inner truths you may previously have been unaware of.

A PATIENT'S STORY

A 57-year-old minister confined to a wheelchair came to see me. We reviewed his health and he told me that he wanted to get off his nightly sleep medications. I gave him some natural remedies that worked for him. At a follow-up visit, I asked him if he was dreaming better, since sleep medicines often affect sleep cycles and dreaming. He said, "In fact, getting off those meds saved my life." I asked him to explain. He had a dream about a mole on his leg and in the dream he was told to check it out. When he woke he made an appointment with a dermatologist. The mole on his leg was removed and found to be early melanoma. "If I hadn't gotten off my sleeping pills, I would have not had this dream and might not have addressed it. So, thank you."

DISCOVER YOUR GIFTS AND PURPOSE

Our health is clearly affected by our attitudes and philosophical beliefs, and our sense of our purpose or life path is an important component. Embracing a spiritual/religious and compassionate view of life is vital to healing and often a source of healing. Asking these philosophical questions we get to our core beliefs about self, and this can also be a powerful way to deal with health issues.

- Who am I?

- Why am I here.

- What is my purpose or mission in life?

- How can I best serve the world?

- Who do I serve?

- What do I have to share with my people and the Earth?

Answering these questions can take a lifetime, and our answers will shift as we grow and change. Give this process time and the right space.

Personally, I feel fortunate to have found my path in life, one that is fulfilling to me. Since my youth I have worked diligently to stay attuned to work, to be open to play, and to change course if guided in that way. I do this by taking time to listen to myself in meditation and by spending time in Nature, and by observing and reflecting on my dreams, a practice that has been quite revealing.

A PERSONAL STORY

My path and passions luckily developed naturally to become a doctor because of my skills, love of learning, and my openness to help, or get close to, people and their lives. After completing medical training, I embraced the studies of many healing systems, which this book represents. These studies of Eastern medicine and philosophy, nutrition, herbal medicine, and mind-body healing also led to my own path of healing, and then doing my first 10-day fast, which transformed me in such positive ways that I started teaching others about it and leading group programs. So, my career path unfolded in ways I consider a part of Taoism, flowing in the river of life, attuned to what feels right in accordance with my inner instincts.

Recently, I experienced a crossroads—should I simplify my clinic and practice to have more time to travel and teach, which is challenging when you oversee and work in a high-overhead, busy medical practice with 20 people? As I tuned in, it was apparent that it wasn't time for me to stop practice because I had many staff, practitioners, and patients counting on me, and since I still felt healthy and strong and liked the patient care part of my life. In fact, I took an even bigger step and commitment by moving the Preventive Medical Center of Marin to new larger space. This process has brought forth a whole new project that my team and I are now experiencing. We are all excited about having a fresh and new practice along with its many challenges and rewards.

Maintaining and progressing an innovative and integrative clinic is an opportunity to make a positive step in my career path. Being a pioneering doctor and creating an example of the NEW Medicine model is part of my life purpose, along with educating people about healthy living, a key part. I hope to continue this for the rest of my days, or as we say at our office, "We'll doc 'til we drop." Hopefully, we will all have many more years.

To reach this connection to purpose may not be easy, and many people need some external guidance, too. What does it take to discover your true self? Sometimes it takes paying the price from injury or illness and recovering from an incident that becomes your guide. For some it comes naturally, while for others it remains a dream while they "work for a living" to support themselves and their family. What's your story?

COMPLETING THE 5 KEYS:
OUR APPROACH TO ILLNESS AND HEALTH

Illnesses can be messages and guides, encouraging us to listen within, learn what the illness and symptoms are saying, and/or determine where they are sending us for healing. Often, there's a message in what our illness prevents us from doing, such as being unable to take a trip, go to a function, stay in a challenging relationship, or keep working at a job we dislike. Thus, our health issues may cause some change in our planned actions, or they may guide us to some new person or treatment. It's important just to be open and receptive to what our body/mind wants. We do this by listening within, which starts with being quiet and breathing, and fully accepting ourselves as who we are and where we are in our lives. No judgments (if possible). With this process, we become more comfortable with our self and develop the ease and courage to 'trust' our instincts and intuition. Learning to relax and meditate enables us to access our inner world's guidance, allowing us to be more peaceful and authentic.

Self-discovery is important at every age. We never stop learning about the effects of our past on our present life and state of health; and we never end the process of learning how to better be who we are. Grandma's wisdom suggests, "Don't worry about your past; correct your future."

"My body is in accord with my mind,
My mind with my energies,
My energies with my spirit..."
—LAO TSU

Embracing these **Five Keys to Staying Healthy** can be a challenge. It may be difficult to give up our favorite "bad" habits, which are those that may be undermining our health without our clear recognition. This may mean taking a coffee break (that's a break from caffeine), a vacation from sugar or alcohol, or trying a gluten-free and/or dairy-free diet. Some of the other challenges may include not activating our life purpose and continuing to feel unfulfilled—and what to do about that.

Ultimately, we are all here to learn, grow, and evolve. When we are clearer within and nourish ourselves well, we may be able to align more with our highest path. Some people, for example, work their entire lives without feeling like they have found their true purpose or used their gifts for the best outcomes. And clearly, most of us do not practice all of these health keys to the best of our abilities all the time. Yet, it helps when seeking to do this and grow as human beings.

To bring all aspects of a healthy lifestyle into a balanced state takes a lot of growth and change, yet change can happen instantaneously, or it can take the tincture of time. The point is to make the changes no matter how long it takes. This is the foundation of health and the place to begin when we are not feeling as well as we would wish or expect. By addressing these key points on a consistent basis, we significantly improve our health both now and in the future.

THE FIVE KEYS SELF SURVEY

How do you rate your Health and Habits in each area?
10 being the best possible

- **Nutrition**   1 – 2 – 3 – 4 – 5 – 6 – 7 – 8 – 9 – 10

- **Exercise**   1 – 2 – 3 – 4 – 5 – 6 – 7 – 8 – 9 – 10

- **Stress**   1 – 2 – 3 – 4 – 5 – 6 – 7 – 8 – 9 – 10

- **Sleep**   1 – 2 – 3 – 4 – 5 – 6 – 7 – 8 – 9 – 10

- **Attitude**   1 – 2 – 3 – 4 – 5 – 6 – 7 – 8 – 9 – 10

Ideally, we are 7 or above in all of these areas.
If not, the low spots are a good place to begin.

Over the years, my patients have responded well to being educated and provided with treatment options other than immediate drug therapy. More specifically, much of this feedback has concerned the changes people have made in their eating and health habits, their exercise, ability to manage stress, and the resulting positive outcomes they have experienced.

TREATMENT OPTIONS

How do we approach illnesses and medical problems when they do occur? We call this the *therapeutic approach*. Often, when we don't feel well, we have a tendency to do what we have been accustomed to doing in the past, or revert back to a Western medicine orientation and attack the problem rather than adopt the Natural medicine approach of first trying to understand and identify its underlying causes, then exploring possible safe, natural solutions.

"LIFESTYLE FIRST, NATURAL THERAPIES NEXT, DRUGS LAST."

This simple maxim is the most sensible approach for both patients and practitioners. However, it may take time, effort and money to discover the underlying lifestyle causes and imbalances at the root of a health problem, and to have guidance and/or know how to rebalance naturally rather than simply treating symptoms with drugs. This approach works most easily for relatively healthy people or during an annual or bi-annual review. Yet, if people are sick, especially with acute illnesses, it may be appropriate to begin therapy with drugs first, and as health improves, transition into more natural therapies and lifestyle corrections. This is a personalized and integrative approach to treating health challenges.

Of course, the goal surrounding any therapy is to get RESULTS, such as eliminating infections, reducing pain, lowering blood pressure, reducing total and "bad" (LDL) cholesterol levels, or clearing allergies. This process involves educating and inviting the patient to be an active partner with their practitioner in the process and progress of the therapy. Examples include daily measurement of blood pressure, weekly tracking of weight and body composition, or conducting a follow-up blood test. Overall, it is wise to follow this approach of "collaborative tracking", since it allows both the patient and practitioner to do the least invasive and least expensive therapies first, unless there's an emergency or life-threatening illness. As Hippocrates reminds us in a primary axiom of medicine, *"First, do no harm."* For ourselves, we may ask, "Do we want to change, or do we have to?"

As we employ this maxim of *Lifestyle First, Natural Therapies Next, and Drugs Last,* we need to ask ourselves, "What can I do to make a difference in my health challenge? Is there some habit or lifestyle activity that may be a contributing factor?" Then, what about any natural remedies? Are there any herbal therapies or a natural program of diet and nutritional supplements that could improve my condition? Or what about mind-body and stress reduction techniques, or structural bodywork? Of course, to answer these questions we will need knowledgeable resources. Natural practitioners, books or reliable sources on the Internet, can be a good place to start. **The more we learn about our body and health, the better self-doctor we can be.**

AN INTEGRATED APPROACH TO TREATING CAUSES

As we have already discovered in chapter 2, one important aspect of NEW Medicine is investigating the underlying causes of illness or disease. It makes sense that by identifying the cause of any problem and addressing that, the problem is likely to recede, or at least be handled more easily when faced with honesty.

Of course, we may not always be successful in this effort. Given the complexity of the human system and the myriad possible causes, some things remain mysterious and are often frustrating and stressful to both patients and practitioners. Many health concerns are referred to as "psychosomatic," meaning they are based in complex mind/body interactions. Yet even with very complex health conditions, I frequently see that through delving deeper, many people can gain insights and help with their conditions, being guided in positive ways to improve their health and even reclaim their optimal health. This may take some new awareness and patience to achieve, as well as some financial support.

> *"Work together to solve and evolve."* —ARGISLE

An integrated approach in healthcare practice begins with looking for causes, understanding the issues in each individual's life, and incorporating multiple systems of healing. Let's clarify what this actually means.

WHAT DEFINES AN INTEGRATED MEDICINE APPROACH?

• **It looks at all aspects of life as they may relate to disease**, not just the current complaints or symptoms of the patient. See what's out of balance, such as why someone would be having a mood or sleep disorder and then finding that they drink two liters of sugared or diet sodas a day. In an integrated program, any combination of lifestyle or areas of personal history could be contributing to the problems for which people seek relief. For example, how long did this symptom take to develop and how did I contribute?

• **It takes a multidisciplinary approach to treatment**. If you as a patient rely only on drug therapy, or as a practitioner, you only have one system that you know, as in Western medicine's use of prescription drugs, this limits the potential for healing more naturally. Exploring and learning to incorporate other strategies and treatments that work to support the healing process is key. As physicians, we might then consider adding other licensed practitioners to support patients.

• **It involves first preventing disease, treating medical conditions, and then sustaining health**. This medical/health experience includes therapeutic support, involving both educational aspects plus other disciplines, such as nutritional guidance, stress management, structural therapies, and general lifestyle motivation. Often, a personal coach for nutrition or exercise at home or in the gym is a great support and motivator for change. Attending local or online workshops and seminars regarding integrative health is also an excellent source of support.

• **It asks different questions about our health and illnesses than conventional medicine**. Rather than "What can I take to make this go away," the new questions, might be "Why is this problem present in my life? Or what's underlying it?" These investigations help us to get to the underlying causes, as discussed above.

CONCLUSION

We have now established the basic principles and practices of NEW Medicine, incorporating Natural, Eastern and Western approaches in a sensible, patient-focused and integrative framework. It feels great to apply many of these healing philosophies that have evolved over hundreds, even thousands, of years in some cases.

While most natural treatments are generally safe and gentle, care should be taken when recommending or using them, since people can have adverse reactions as well (although this is quite uncommon). Also, natural therapies like herbal remedies do not always act quickly against acute problems, and they often require more time to create results than do many drugs. Eastern medicine approaches are generally safe and soothing/relaxing, yet these treatments also take time and require great art on the part of the practitioner to be administered effectively. Western medicine can be strong and often rapid in its effects. Yet as we know, drugs can often result in toxicity, side effects, and possible addictions and expense.

The principles and precautions presented here highlight the fact that it is essential to know and apply the best approaches to achieve optimal outcomes for each patient'. unique health needs. We can apply some of the Natural, Eastern or Western modalities individually or in a combination. Of course, it is wisest to use the simplest and safest treatment that will work for you.

In summary, here are five positive affirmations that I use myself and that you might consider bringing into your life. Which ones seem important to you? Maybe create your own.

Five Keys—Five Affirmations

1. I eat to nourish myself

I try to make good choices about what I consume, yet, I also get to enjoy some of my favorite treats on occasion. I avoid creating any unsupportive daily habits with substances like sugar, caffeine, alcohol, or nicotine. If I am challenged with these or other health-undermining eating habits, I work to free myself from them.

2. I find my best and most balanced exercise.

I see the results, and enjoy the process. Consistency is important. Balance means a mix of stretching for flexibility, weights for strength, aerobic activity for endurance, and all leads to feeling good, staying lighter and more relaxed. I avoid sitting around and being too lazy, yet I also need to rest. I exercise with the seasons and this allows me to continue and adjust my fitness program year around.

3. I learn to relax, meditate, and clear my anxieties and fears.

I remain clear, strong and energized without being over stimulated. I turn my faith over to the higher forces of spirit. I take things in stride and know the universe offers me challenges as opportunities to learn and grow. I also practice my people skills and learn how both to get along as well as disagree with others without aggression.

4. I learn to sleep like a baby

I know that good sleep is central to my health so I pay attention to my sleep hygiene and keep my nighttime electromagnetic (EMFs) stress exposures low. Prioritize sleep and make sure you rest and recharge nightly as you are able. If needed, use relaxation techniques and natural remedies before turning to prescription sleeping pills.

5. I maintain an attitude of gratitude

Every day I express my love and appreciation of myself (and others close to me), knowing that if I treat my body in a positive and loving way, I will more likely Stay Healthy.

Personal Review: Healthy Living Guidelines

Let's review all we have talked about by embracing the many aspects of a healthy lifestyle while being attentive to our daily choices and activities. Use some of these health philosophies while staying connected to yourself.

- **KNOW YOURSELF.**

  Begin by looking within—using meditation and listening to your deeper self. What do you do with your personal time, your leisure time? What do you do based on your health intuition and inner guidance? Do you even have health intuition, or do you count on your health practitioner to tell you everything?

- **WHAT NEEDS TO BE CHANGED?**

  What are the best healing habits to develop for your health, your connection to others, and the Earth? Which ones are most important for you? Choose three, and do this after you look at your life and habits, and sense what issues may be undermining your health the most. What changes can (and will) you make now?

- **HOW DO YOU EAT?**

  Plan your food intake and follow through instead of going with cravings and treats when you are hungry. Eat mostly fresh foods and plenty of vegetables—50% by volume for most people as suggested in my book, *More Vegetables, Please!* Making weekly menu plans, shopping lists and recipes you want to try will help you to follow a healthy, balanced diet.

- **MOVE MORE**

  Create and actually do a balanced exercise program that includes stretching for flexibility, weight training for strength, and aerobic activity for endurance as well as sweating to support body/mind detoxification. Walk when you can, or bike instead of driving, but ideally not on busy city streets where our exposure to gasoline fumes are a concern.

- **DETOX**

  Benefit from regular detoxification programs based on body type, lifestyle and personal needs—as important as taking a vacation from work. Twice a year is a good basic plan, ideally in the Spring and Autumn.

- **REST, RELAX, and SLEEP**
Adequate sleep, deep rest and relaxation are key to Staying Healthy and Energetic.

- **STRESS LESS**
Manage stress and emotions to stay in balance and at peace, while keeping your goals and motivation alive—this means also staying in touch with your feelings.

- **COOPERATE and CONNECT**
Learn how to both cooperate and healthfully disagree with loved ones and co-workers without causing blame and resentment. Hopefully, they want this as well.

- **COMMUNICATE CLEARLY**
Maintain healthy relationships and open lines of communications with all important family, friends, and co-workers. If you have trouble expressing yourself easily, take a class on this or get some help from a professional.

- **TUNE IN**
Attune to your needs and cycles, and plan what health therapies are right for you. Massage, acupuncture or making and taking special time to nourish and support your being, are essential to maintaining good health.

- **GROW IN EVERY WAY**
Plant a garden, grow some of your own food, and stay connected to the Earth. Use pots and trays on your deck or windowsill if you don't have a garden. Get your hands in the dirt. Also, be open to learn new things and embrace life with passion and presence, because growth and evolution are keys to a healthy and long life with vitality.

- **REMEMBER TO BE**
You are not a human doing, but primarily a human being. Take time to be, with yourself and others, and take quiet time also to rest and meditate so you have clarity from your inner sanctum.

- **LOVE YOURSELF**
My personal motto of recent years is "Keep love in my heart all day, say YES whenever I can, and be able to say NO." It all starts with our hearts and being our authentic selves.

CHAPTER 4

THE DOCTOR-PATIENT RELATIONSHIP
The Basis for Healing

Now that the key health principles of NEW Medicine have been discussed, let's explore important aspects of the primary relationship of health care, the one between the patient and the physician. The doctor-patient relationship (DPR) is central to an effective healing system for each person. Let's also explore important qualities to seek the kind of medical practice and practitioner we (and our family and finances) select for our care. We have choices in discovering the best medical situation for us. How can we be assured of conscious and conscientious care within a medical practice? Most of us require guidance and education to embrace healthier lifestyle practices and natural approaches, helping us improve our conditions and prevent future health challenges where possible.

When first becoming a doctor, I realized that understanding what constitutes good medical care was much more than mere knowledge; it also involved motivation, insight, sensitivity and application of safe and helpful treatments. Creating an effective practice for the people who come to see me—reaching out and really connecting with people—is aligned with being the best, most effective practitioner and healer for my patients and for myself. At the outset, I asked myself, "How can I inspire my patients to take better care of themselves, and keep my own health strong as well?" As a young doctor, I believed (and still do) that so many health problems are the result of unhealthy lifestyle habits, plus a lack of health education and health support about the basics of caring for the human body and the environment—both from parents, families, friends and schools. Much of what we need is just good old common sense, applying the basic principles on a consistent basis.

> ### RISK—BENEFIT
>
> When considering any treatment, assess all options, such as efficacy, risks and costs, with the understanding that longer lasting health typically occurs when that treatment fits within the mutual belief systems of the practitioner and the patient, which can easily affect the physical and mental outcomes.

The first step in a personally successful DPR is to identify what's important to you in a relationship with your physician/practitioner so that you are engaged and excited to maintain your health and wellness, while also making certain that you can afford it. There may be one individual or a team of practitioners that fit your needs and beliefs.

The relationship between healer and patient has existed since the beginning of human interactions and the delineation of certain roles among tribe members. For thousands of years, this was a sacred and trusted bond. However, with the advent of technology and fast-paced medical care, this relationship has changed, and some might say it has become less personal and more procedural. It has also led to increased levels of specialization and less focus on general medical care and family health. Such changes are also driven by the increased demands upon modern practitioners by insurance companies to limit the time spent and to treat more and more patients. Yet, in spite of the forces and changes that depersonalize the DPR, today there still exists a special pact between doctor/healer and patient, with increasing possibilities of regaining many positive aspects of future, healthier bonds. Now let's look at relevant, specific interactions between doctors and patients and explore how to improve this essential relationship.

QUALITIES OF A HEALTHY DOCTOR-PATIENT RELATIONSHIP

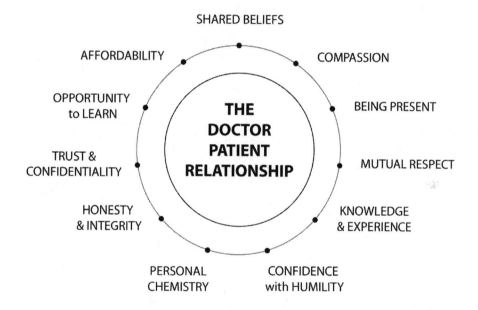

Many qualities and elements factor into a quality DPR. My list of priorities may be different than yours. **What qualities top your list?** Are trust and respect foremost? Or is it your doctor's level of knowledge and experience, or perhaps logistics such as easy access at a convenient location, simplicity in making appointments, or what your insurance covers? Financial resources play a significant role for most patients who might tolerate a lesser quality DPR that is more affordable. Here are the qualities that I deem important and relevant for a good relationship.

SHARED BELIEFS

An ideal DPR involves an alignment of belief systems between the doctor and patient enabling them to work together successfully to achieve common goals. Doctors and healers should be supportive of our experiences and beliefs, even when they don't agree with or understand them completely. Conversely, a patient searching for alternative practices will likely be open to new approaches and ideas from a trusted healer. While each practitioner knows about his or her own field, he or she may know little about other systems of medicine not taught in medical school that the patient may be using or considering as potential options. For example, when going to a Western doctor for an evaluation and treatment, be open to diagnostic tests, medical treatments and/or a pharmaceutical prescription. Of course we, have the right to choose to follow this recommendation or not (referred to as *adherence to treatment*). What is important is that the doctor and patent have a trusted understanding, coupled with an ability to discuss matters openly and determine the best course for diagnosis and treatment, along with awareness of expenses for any treatment, as well as time, cost, potential effectiveness and impact on loved ones.

Adherence (or non-adherence) is important for continuity of care and is the consequence when patients follow through with agreed-upon therapies or taking their prescribed medications. For example, sometimes, patients are skeptical and fearful of Western drug therapies, or they simply can't afford them. At this point in the DPR, there can be a disconnect between what the doctor has recommended as the best treatment for the patient, and what the patient is actually doing. Is the patient "adhering," or have they changed course without informing their doctor. Not taking a prescribed medication represents one clear example of a failed "shared beliefs" relationship, and it may relate to finances.

Researchers at Harvard Medical School published the largest study to date of what has been termed "primary non-adherence" and found that more than 20% of first-time patient prescriptions were never filled, and overall, nearly half the patients took their drugs as prescribed.[1] A more recent study from NYU Medical School found that African-American patient adherence for taking the prescribed high blood pressure medications was better when the patient was given health education and even better after learning about positive thoughts and affirmations.[2]

A first level of care involves the process of collaboration between patient and doctor. Occasionally people visit a doctor asking for a certain prescription and/or certain testing; In my case, I give them every opportunity to voice such requests, and support them even if it means putting my own personal beliefs aside. I listen without judging, or making them feel wrong, and do not dismiss their feelings, views or belief systems—this would show disrespect, which is not part of a healthy DPR. If, however, after listening and considering the patient's requests, their choices seem to be either incorrect or potentially harmful, I will also respectfully suggest an alternative treatment choice which they may not know about.

If a patient requests a treatment that I have little or no experience in providing, I refer them to someone more appropriate. For example, when a patient's request is for medicines or tests or procedures that I haven't used or evaluated for effectiveness and risk, I explain my position and then may refer them to another practitioner with more experience in these matters. There are occasions where instead of referring to another practitioner, I will research to learn more about the topic in question. Or I may call known specialists and ask their opinion and guidance in regard to testing, treatment or referral. These are many ways that patients and doctors can learn and grow together. I may share my personal approach and thinking, about their condition and the treatment recommended. This is how to create a collaborative environment and respect. Most of all, patients want their doctor to be honest, helpful and straightforward with their information and not be unaware, insensitive, or in a rush.

INTEGRATIVE, MULTIDISCIPLINARY CARE

There is more than one way to treat people medically, and many natural therapies account for the wide variety of patient needs and belief systems. I have expanded my treatment options in other areas besides prescriptive medicines. These are the "N" for Natural and "E" for Eastern aspects of NEW Medicine. Many patients want safer, yet effective and more natural ways of treatment for their medical problems, or even more importantly, for balancing or preventing illnesses in the first place. Lifestyle change clearly plays a major role in preventing disease; still, many patients go to see a Western doctor because that is where they usually go for their medical care and what is typically covered by insurance.

ALIGNED CHOICES

It is important for both doctor and patient to consider all available and possible options in regard to a given medical or health issue. There is a saying, *"To a hammer, everything looks like a nail."* Most doctors would state, "I do what I am trained to do." For example, if you go to a surgeon to address a health issue, it is likely that you may have surgery recommended as your primary or at least one of your options. This is, of course, an appropriate choice if your body really needs surgical repair. However, what if a simpler medical or even natural, approach may allow you to postpone or even avoid surgery? It is advisable for patients to investigate the belief system or practice philosophy of their healthcare providers in advance, either by calling the office or reviewing on the Internet. You can also reach out and talk to other post-surgery patients. Taking these important steps at the outset greatly increases the probability of a positive DPR and desired outcome, while unnecessary testing, surgery, prescriptions and other therapies may be avoided, along with the stress of the additional expenses.

Most Western doctors have been trained to be quick, decisive and authoritative—which can be advantageous when making decisions that are both correct and with which you concur, or when there is a crisis situation demanding an immediate response. These qualities can clearly save lives. Yet, most medical situations are not crises and immediate decisions do not need to be made "on the spot.. Often, there are many complex factors to consider about a patient's health and need for healing, some of which become evident over time and with considerable interaction between the Doctor and Patient. It is important that your doctor knows how to be thoughtful, caring and willing to take the take the time to make the wisest decisions. Ultimately, your health is not about a "quick fix," but rather about a long-term transition to optimal healthy and vital outcomes.

If you decide to seek care from an Eastern Medicine practitioner/acupuncturist you will likely have your lifestyle, habits, and imbalances reviewed, and you should be open to acupuncture treatments, dietary and lifestyle changes, and herbal therapies. Or you may decide to seek care from a Western herbalist or naturopath, which will involve their philosophies and treatment approaches, such as hands-on body care, a dietary change, or a light cleansing program (if that's right for you), plus an array of appropriate nutritional and herbal supplements. Many patients seek care from a variety of Natural, Eastern, and Western healthcare providers, involving alignment of choices between each care provider and the patient. As you select your healthcare provider it is important to know your own personal goals and philosophy about your health and healing—this optimizes the possibility for identifying the best healthcare providers and creating the optimal DPR with your health as CEO.

The ever-increasing specialization in medicine tends to restrict patient care to one area of health instead of seeing the bigger picture of total health and wellness. For example, Cardiovascular Disease (CVD) is one of the leading medical problems. Often, the primary option offered to a patient with angina from blocked arteries in the heart, which is a consequence of CVD and a serious concern, is a surgical bypass procedure (or the placement of stents to open the arteries). It is one of the most common major elective surgical procedures in the US, UK, and Australia.[3] Obviously, the coronary artery bypass surgery may fix the end result problem of clogged arteries, but it doesn't address the underlying process and often the procedure needs to be repeated years later. Also after successful bypass surgery, the resulting emotional states, such as anxiety and depression, must be addressed for best results.[4] Clearly, there should be a discussion of medical management options before such a major procedure is undertaken, along with education about the effects of diet, exercise, and stress management on the CVD recovery and therapeutic process. Many cardiologists and family physicians do this in their offices themselves or with staff. This type of treatment may involve prescription medicines, nutritional supplements, detoxification, stress reduction, diet and lifestyle changes—all of which cost less, are non-invasive, avoid pain and recovery time, and help restore some of the function of the cardiovascular system as well as often improve overall health. However, when comparing medical evidence, many long-term studies looked primarily at life and death rather than improved quality of life or the correction of the underlying causes. In many instances the results of medical treatment (primarily pharmaceutical) for CVD are often equivalent or even superior to surgery. In many health conditions, approaches involving natural therapies and nutritional counseling—when applied at the right time (typically the earlier the better)—may offer more positive results and lower costs than drugs and surgery[5]. Another aspect of comparing evidence of outcomes is that drug and procedural processes that are patentable will have more money available to them for research while natural treatments may in fact, lack many financial resources to be tested properly (so far!).

> Dean Ornish, MD has developed a very successful program to treat cardiovascular disease. His research has shown that lifestyle and dietary changes, plus exercise, stress management, and emotional counseling not only helps to prevent cardiovascular disease, but also to reverse the disease in patients[6]. Of course, each case is unique and requires individual attention and mutual decisions between doctor and patient. More research with positive lifestyle changes would likely show positive outcomes for many health conditions. This would be especially true when both the healthcare practitioner and patient are aligned and cooperate toward a similar healing result. Motivation and adherence to a program's steps and stages are keys to its success. Ornish's initial lifestyle intervention was for 30 days with cardiac benefits lasting one year and subsequent studies indicated more and longer lasting results.[7]

Usually there is not a single "right answer" for treating most medical conditions. Remember, it's called medical *practice*, because in essence, that's what doctors do; they are constantly trying to perfect the system of diagnosis and treatment for their patients. Although we may laugh when we say we are practicing, the fact is that the art and science of medicine is a dynamic process within an ever changing and expanding field of health care. And each patient is an individual and needs special and appropriate care.

COMPASSION & CARE

Compassion and caring—the true "heart of healing"—are too often missing from today's frenzied healthcare system. These qualities sincerely expressed by a healthcare provider, help patients feel that there is genuine concern and a deep commitment to the healing process, coupled with empathy with the conditions and struggles being faced. In the healing paradigm, research suggests that it is the quality of relationship and finding common ground[8] that makes a difference in the patient's adherence[9] and recovery.[10] When there is an absence of compassion, trust and care, patients tend to feel more isolated and disconnected, making the healing process less effective and often more costly. Yet, from a physician's point of view, there also needs to be a certain degree of detachment from patients, since getting too close, or feeling too emotionally involved, may alter the essential process of objective decision-making. This is why many doctors elect to not treat their immediate family members, or themselves. Thus, creating the right balance of attentiveness and listening along with loving kindness and authentic caring goes a long way.

PATIENT-CENTERED CARE AND CONCIERGE MEDICINE

Patient-centered care is a common term for practices that really cater to the patient and their needs, and to the communications between physician and patient. This might be called "collaborative care" with the patient contributing to decisions. My clinic motto is, "Serve people with the best quality care." Often this can be within the insurance model, yet some doctors and practices use a Concierge Medicine model, charging extra (sometimes a yearly fee) to provide additional or "high-priority" care to enrolled patients. Such enhancements might include same-day appointments or callbacks, Internet availability, office educational programs, and so on.

Research suggests that both of these models may help improve patients' health and provide more efficient care utilizing less diagnostic tests or specialist referrals.[11] This is a wave of the future for some advancement in health care to make for deeper relationships with the medical practices and patients.

Of course, not everyone wishes to choose these services and the additional fees, whether a yearly membership or month-to-month charges, ranging from a couple hundred dollars to thousands per year. This is great if it's affordable, but the question is, why can't everyone get this kind of service? Simply, most doctors have too many patients with too many needs to provide this more extensive individualized care to everyone. That's why there is the additional charge—it allows doctors to have less patients and less stress in providing additional care.

A primary focus of Western medical training has been to teach doctors to fix things and respond to pain and suffering much like a mechanic. Yet, in spite of our best medical efforts, many aches and pains or illnesses take time to resolve. I often say, "It's a lucky thing that many symptoms and conditions get better on their own (in time); otherwise the physicians' reputation may not be worthy of the trust we already may have." 'Let things be, watch and see' is important in the right situations unless of course, there is a clear urgency or emergency.

> As a parent, I learned more about empathy and care, and it helped me get over the need to fix everything right away. My children's mother, Tara, who has good psychological insights (and is a practicing hypnotherapist), coached me when our kids were young and occasionally unwell. Rather than just trying to fix a problem, she suggested first saying to them, "I'm sorry that you don't feel well, or are in pain (as the case may be)." This compassionately connects you and is a good start, plus it helps as a dad and as a doctor as well. Yet as physicians, we also want to identify solutions and help when that is possible and desired; doctors are trained to intervene and act. Overall, it's important to show you care and to also show at some level that you understand the person and their problem. Many illnesses are self-limited; in other words, they get better on their own.

THE POWER OF THE PLACEBO

Compassion can have quite a positive effect upon the healing process. The placebo effect was originally defined as a clinical response following the patient receiving an inactive substance or a sham treatment. Can a fake antibiotic heal an infection? Can anything be healing if the body/mind believes it?

The term *placebo* has evolved to reflect the fact that the person's self-healing mechanism[12] has been turned on - a process called "the Meaning Response."[13] The placebo effect is based on the individual's beliefs and internal biology that affect the improvement or change.[14] The doctor's beliefs may also play a role here. However, we are still not clear about the actual mechanism of the placebo response; it may have something to do with a good DPR, but more than likely it is related to the patient's core beliefs about healing and illness. There's also a phenomenon called the "nocebo" effect, the process where negative thoughts and images contribute to negative results, such as with people experiencing drug reactions and side effects.

Shared Beliefs, Common Ground, and Confidence in both the practitioner and the treatment can create what's called **Positive Imagery** that may also enhance the healing (or placebo) potential of any therapy. This involves the supportive use of words (ambiance, caring, touch, and more—the whole experience) by practitioners creating a positive image/idea for the patient's healing. Once you decide to use any treatment, BELIEVE that it will work. Doctors need to encourage patients to believe in what they do, and patients can be asking and guiding their physicians to be supportive with their words so as to not undermine the treatment and the overall DPR.

BEING PRESENT & CONNECTING

Patients want a doctor who pays attention, is focused on them and listens; in other words, one who is fully present. These are good qualities for every practitioner, also for any person in relationships with others, be they personal or professional. When the doctor isn't fully engaged and doesn't hear your concern or get to know you, how effective can he or she be in assessing your health condition and developing a treatment plan? Like any serious relationship, getting to know one another requires time for both doctors and patients. It's an investment in Staying Healthy, no matter your challenges.

> A combined Canadian and US study found that doctors interrupted their patients on average within 23 seconds from the time the patient begins explaining his symptoms.[15] In 25% of visits, the doctor never even asked the patients what was bothering them. Somehow a typical doctor's visit has been defined as fifteen minutes.[16] In another study that taped 34 physicians during more than 300 visits with patients, the doctors spent on average 1.3 minutes conveying crucial information about the patient's condition and treatment, and most of the information they provided was far too technical for the average patient to grasp; disconcertingly, those same doctors thought they had spent more than eight minutes. In another study, three out of four doctors failed to give clear instructions on how to take medication. When asked to state medication instructions, half of patients have no idea what they are supposed to do.[17]

The continuity, quality, and duration of sessions between doctor and patient have direct bearings on the quality of the DPR, for better or worse. A big issue is the length of visits patients have with doctors, and especially with long waits. As with many parts of our present healthcare system, such as urgent care or with an HMO, patients often see different doctors each time they have an appointment (in recent years this has been improving with Kaiser and other HMOs), or the doctors change jobs more frequently resulting in higher turnover and less continuity with patients. These aspects of our current healthcare system cannot be avoided, but they can be minimized.

The basis and growth of a good DPR begins when doctors and patients know each other over the years and cycles of their lives, as with our old style "family doctor." There is clearly a difference in the quality of the relationship when there are many visits and inter-actions over time. This creates a connectedness that builds trust and alignment. Of course, Americans are a highly mobile society with the average American moving every five years.[18] Continuity of care becomes even more problematic, as well as jobs and/or insur-ance coverage may change and this leads people to seek other docs approved by their plans.

MAKING IT PERSONAL

A positive aspect of family medicine, which is being lost in part to spe-cialties, is the long-term relationships with patients and getting to know them and their lives. Seeing other family members adds to this deeper relationship, as does seeing their parents or children. In working with lifestyle remodeling as a way to change health outcomes, it really helps to have the spouse (and children) involved so that everyone in the household is on board for different diets, exercise programs and even handling stress and emotional issues.

A physician being present, listening and taking time, plus when a doctor shows attentive care not only about what's going on with you, but also about who you are as a person, your work and your family, may all result in a better give-and-take interchange. Being in the same office for 30 years provides a rewarding part of prac-tice—I've seen people regularly and know about their families, seeing them for a healthy check-up and check-in five or ten years after their previous visit. This is how some healthy people choose to use our system, as their own "health watch," working together to maintain their body's balance. These same people might also see an acupuncturist, chiropractor or massage therapist for their health maintenance. Of course, as part of a healthy DPR, each practitioner should know about all the other practitioners their patient sees and the treatments they are receiving.

MUTUAL RESPECT

Vital to any healthy DPR is mutual respect. In medical school, this was sorely lacking, and I came to realize over the years that this is an endemic weakness of our Western Medical system-- not treating patients as human beings first and honoring them for their feelings, concerns and their time. In *The Health Bill of Rights* (see end of chapter) we review the issues of respect for each other's time and human medical rights, with personal respect for one another as human beings. These rights also relate to complex questions such as belief systems and practical matters such as not keeping patients waiting for many hours. Maybe we should suggest that patients bill their doctors for waiting time, or at least offer something special.

As a doctor, I honor you and seek to do the best I can to help and support you. After all, that is the core service of the medical "helping" profession, and this is a primary reason why patients go to doctors or other health practitioners in the first place—to seek help, get clear insights and solutions regarding their condition, to ease pain and suffering, to receive guidance for personal dilemmas, emotional frustrations and even to seek relief for common problems such as fatigue and insomnia.

Respect is a two-way street, and for doctors to respect patients is only half of the equation. As patients, it is our role to be respectful and supportive of the practice policies, the staff and the doctor's time. It really helps to understand these parameters before even going to a practitioner the first time. We should endeavor to find out what is expected from us. Are there forms that need to be filled out before we go in for an appointment? Do we understand the costs and insurance coverage if that is relevant, etc.? We can always call the office or go to the website to find out the basic information before we make an appointment or visit the practice. Eventually, you find out if it's a good fit. Is the office a healthy place and is the staff healthy and supportive?

My goal is to be on time as much as possible; so we don't double book patients to protect the bottom line in case of no-shows; each person has a specific place in my schedule. Timing is thrown off when people are late or when new patients don't have all their forms completed. Then I feel a bit rushed to get through the issues at hand, or I may not be able to cover all the medical/health concerns and must focus on the key needs. This also affects all the patients with scheduled appointments for the rest of the day; thus **it takes everyone involved to make the practice work effectively**. When doctors honor and respect their patients, and when patients are respectful of the doctor, staff and practice, there is a major improvement in health outcomes, the DPR and the overall healthcare system.

"The good physician treats the disease; the great physician treats the patient who has the disease. It is much more important to know what sort of a patient has a disease than what sort of a disease a patient has."
—WILLIAM OSLER, MD (1849-1919), *Pioneer Of Modern Medicine*

THE WAITING GAME:
PART OF PATIENT DISATISFACTION

One of the biggest patient complaints about doctors is waiting for appointments, both in scheduling and when actually being at the doctor's office. Has this happened to you? As an example, your appointment card may say 2 PM and you arrive on time to a waiting room full of patients, Yet, it may be 3-4 PM before you are actually called and placed in a room to wait some more, since many doctors have three to four treatment rooms they move through to see their patients. Finally, at 4:30 PM your doctor comes in, surely aware that he or she is late and maybe/hopefully apologizes. Yet, that is little comfort since she or he is clearly rushed, leaving you to feel badly about asking the questions you may have about your condition, concerns, future treatment plans, etc. Being upset is not a path to healing. These visits are important to each patient—usually it is the only such visit that day or week, and each patient's individual health hinges upon the outcome. But to many doctors, that visit is one of many, perhaps too many. Ultimately, it has taken the patient 3-4 hours for a 5-10 minute visit (if that long) with the doctor. This may be less common than in the past, yet it still happens too often. Many people state that they feel disrespected, unattended to and overcharged from their visits to doctors, and this is exacerbated when they also wait too long. In the US, waiting also comes down to getting an appointment with your physician. One criticism about socialized medicine or universal care is the long wait for a doctor's appointment. The Commonwealth Fund compared wait times in the US to 10 other countries. In that study, 26% of American adults waited six days or more, which was worse than countries with national health systems; in the UK, only 16% of adults had to wait more than 6 days.[19]

Of course, every doctor and practice has their own scheduling and time issues, which can vary widely depending upon the size and type of the practice. For example, 5-10 minutes may be more than enough office time for a dermatologist observing a skin rash or examining a mole and doing a simply biopsy, whereas the wait to see the dermatologist could be anywhere from 14-72 days depending on which city you were in.[20] An endocrinologist, on the other hand, may require more time (20-30 minutes or more) to sort out symptoms and evaluate hormonal balance and imbalance, review or order lab tests, and understand a patient's needs by tuning in more to the specific situation. Of course, these factors vary among doctors and some people have more complex health issues. In a recent survey of 1000 Americans, what bothered them the most after their doctor's visit was unclear explanations of their problem. The second most common complaint was long waiting times in either the waiting or exam rooms.[21]

MESSAGE TO PHYSICIANS

I implore all my medical colleagues to be more respectful of their patients' time. That means understanding first how you work, how many people you can really see, and for how long; then schedule them accordingly. I understand that there needs to be a few extras scheduled to balance 'no-shows' and to satisfy the patients who require more care as well as to keep the schedule full. I am sure that both you and your patients will appreciate this. Also, many practices charge for late cancelled appointments and no-shows. Yet, do we compensate people for their time away from work or family when we keep them waiting? Fairness is key to a healthy DPR too.

HEALTHY EXAMPLES

Physicians are legally the leaders in their private practices. It's a benefit for them to set a good example for health and wellness. When we care for ourselves and support our staff to do the same through their education and growth, we serve as tangible examples of bringing more health into our practice. Healthcare professionals and their support staff should recognize that their own health and wellbeing are pre-requisites to delivering optimal care and supporting health to others. In our present system of crisis care, the "health of the healers" is not made a priority, and little is done to encourage physical health and stress reduction for those often in greatest need. A change here would improve our entire healthcare system. In general, nurses and medical assistants are stressed, with much expected of them, especially in the hospital setting.

THE HEALTH OF THE HEALERS

There is profound truth in the adage, *"Physician, Heal Thyself."* Without health among our nation's healers, how can we truly and effectively serve patients' needs. Moreover, in the context of modern health care in the US today, the requirement for true "health-of-the healer" extends well-beyond individual healthcare practitioners, since it is actually the entire medical practice that administers healing solutions to patients.

KNOWLEDGE & EXPERIENCE

In a healthy DPR, patients also look for knowledge and experience, which is directly correlated with an increase in confidence and trust of the patient for and with the doctor. Most practitioners, especially medical doctors and other licensed professionals, learn a great deal of their trade over years of study and guidance by experienced teachers before they are able to begin practicing on their own. When a doctor's education and knowledge are complemented by high levels of professionalism, respectfulness and care, the DPR is successful, even if the doctor hasn't been in practice for twenty years or more. Experience matters most with more complicated medical problems and this often involves more specialized training and treatments. In modern medicine, we have specialists in endo-crinology, orthopedics, cardiology, and every area of the body and mind. Thus, there are situations when a patient's problem seems out of a primary care doctor's comfort zone or experience. However, most general and family practitioners know the basics of these areas of health care and can handle most common problems with mutual cooperation when needed.

Often, during challenging times of illness, a patient is sent from place to place, filling out form after form, and having varied approaches sug-gested if they are seeing different specialists or types of practitioners. This can add further stress to their potentially fragile emotional state.

Experience comes from years of study and work (and sometimes by learning from the mistakes we all make). It is essential that practi-tioners don't become jaded, bitter or aloof. We all need to be human first, expressing the qualities of any good relationship. While many physicians and practitioners have training in one or more special-ties, a good doctor needs to go beyond the mechanics of any spe-cific training, giving rise to the maxim in medical school for each procedure. "Show one, do one, teach one." They also need to be able to think clearly and at times expansively and "outside the box" to address patient's real issues and still do what it takes to clearly address health issues in an affordable and timely manner. You can see that so much is required to restore and nourish people with good care that becomes effective because the patient is receptive.

What about intuition? This gift allows us to experience, feel, or see more subtle or invisible levels of people, their situations and their health. Since good medicine is really an art as much as a science, it's helpful when a practitioner appreciates and uses their "sixth sense," and this can be helpful in making good choices and decisions. Each of us is intuitive when we practice seeing the subtle aspects of ourself and address what's living inside us. As we reviewed in Chapter 3, it's valuable to be attuned to our soul essence and our individual purpose on Earth—who we are at the core.

OPEN MINDEDNESS TO OTHER APPROACHES

It is essential for doctor and patient to be open to all possible approaches to achieve healing and optimal health. Ideally practitioners focus first on what is best for the patient—not on their own practice—and as mentioned, this may result in referring the patient to another practitioner. While in the short term, this may not benefit a practitioner, it is certainly best for the patient and ultimately the practitioner, in becoming more trusted and respected to serve the patient.

Question doctors about their level of openness to other approaches, and ask if they ever determined that they were possibly not the best fit for a patient's needs. In collaboration, it is also essential that patients bring an open mind to the relationship as they develop a commitment to working in the process of a healthy DPR. Biases toward one approach versus another may not be in the patient's best interest—this is where trust in the doctor and respect for the many years of education and experience come in.

A clinic with a variety of practitioners supports a wider range of knowledge and experience than a solo practice. To treat patients only with a single skill set or specialty may or may not be sufficient, and may require sending an ill and vulnerable person here, there and everywhere to seek healing. Will this be doing more harm than good?

People are already too busy these days with too many demands, places to go, and things to do. Since doctors and clinics are service organizations, why not provide high-quality service? We are not here to create more stress. Thus, in my practice we have endeavored to build a complementary team of knowledgeable practitioners so that we may respond to a variety of needs and opportunities to serve our patients. This multidisciplinary approach takes "knowledge and experience" to the next level!

"You treat a disease, you win or you lose. You treat a person, I guarantee you, you'll win, no matter what the outcome."

—HUNTER "PATCH" ADAMS, MD

CONFIDENCE WITH HUMILITY

Patients prefer doctors to be confident and "know their stuff," yet who are not arrogant, which creates distance for any relationship. Also, many patients feel that good practitioners should also be respectful and open to listen and learn from their patients, and be willing and able to talk at a level that the patient understands. Thus, **confidence and humility** go together well in a healthy DPR. When patients aren't feeling well, they are particularly vulnerable, and may have difficulties dealing with the extra stress of an insensitive doctor. It is important that the practitioner realizes that words and tone can have great impact upon a patient's mental and emotional wellbeing, and ultimately the patient's health outcome. Exhibiting a friendly, comforting demeanor, while also communicating confidence, works well to support a vulnerable or ill patient and optimizes the probability of a good DPR and successful outcome.

PATIENT CONCERNS ABOUT AUTHORITY

Many patients come to see me—sometimes in tears—describing what other doctors have told them and how they were belittled or treated with disrespect. These patients experienced what they felt were insensitive and overly authoritative doctor-patient encounters. Some were threatened with a bad outcome if the doctor's advice was not followed, creating an additional element of anxiety and fear. Not surprisingly, many doctors focus on diagnosis, pronouncing outcomes and statistical projections about certain conditions or treatments that fit within their belief system and research, supporting and reinforcing their views. They may be right or wrong in these particular circumstances. Is this an example of the doctor "playing God," or just being the authoritative expert depending on the best current research? Even if they are correct, you may seek further counsel before a decision is made. Statistical projections mean that a certain percentage of people will respond positively to a particular protocol and some won't (no approach works 100% of the time). This didactic and dominating approach to health care is important for life-and-death situations and emergencies, yet most health situations and decisions do not fit into these categories, and are better served when the doctor and patient enter into a real dialogue, with shared respect and trust, along with clarifying any costs and timelines. When practitioners dismiss their patients' ideas, or other systems of medical care (besides their own), they may upset or offend some patients, breaking the DPR bond of trust. Many patients appreciate a doctor taking time to consider alternative, complementary approaches to their health concerns, listening to and respecting the patient. This is a more constructive way to investigate the possibilities of treatment and strengthen the DPR. Both need to discover if they are on the same page with regards to philosophy of healing approaches, and expected outcomes, finances and time.

*I feel blessed to do what I do, and privileged to have been educated in an array of healthcare traditions and practices—both ancient and modern—and to have practiced these for decades to gain the experience and confidence to offer my patients. I also feel blessed to have created close bonds with many people (and staff) over the years, and am able to put myself in their place for a moment, gaining insights to come up with solutions for (often with them) when able. I am humbled and honored daily and one of the major reasons for taking care of myself is to insure that I feel and have positive energy to offer, and that I am a good example of the health philosophy I embrace. Keeping fit and healthy is crucial for modeling for our patients, especially when we as doctors are so exposed to many ill patients. Thus, **confidence and humility go heart-in-hand with a quality practitioner.***

PERSONAL CHEMISTRY

Personal chemistry is unique to every relationship; sometimes we "click" and sometimes we don't. The right relationships and friends is important for all of us as part of leading a fulfilling life and able to be of greatest service. Yet—as with our family or work associates—we don't always have a choice about who we live or work with, and sometimes these relationships can be particularly challenging. In a medical setting, it can be similar to an HMO physician who is "assigned" to a patient without that patient's consent or input. In such cases, patients learn to cope and heal as best they can. Luckily, in most cases we can either choose or change practitioners when we are dissatisfied. This is a clear case when you, the patient, have an active role in improving your part of the DPR.

Positive personal chemistry is critical to a healthy DPR. As physicians, every patient we see is not necessarily a good match. A given patient's needs or expectations may not fit with what we know or what we have to offer. Even when we care about people and want to help them, often we just can't. Sometimes personalities clash or the medical problems may be too complex and we don't have the answers. We must be able to recognize discordances that can impact the DPR, knowing that not all doctor-patient pairings offer the best fit. In such cases we need to refer the patient to someone who can supply expertise. On the other hand, great and satisfying health care can come from good chemistry; this includes enhanced trust, confidence, and openness to alternative approaches, plus willingness to commit the time and energy needed for true healing.

DPR AND HEALTH OUTCOMES

Lack of adequate time and the complexity of care have left the doctor-patient relationship in tatters. And this makes a huge difference in patient care. Numerous studies have found a link between how well the doctor and patient communicate and the patient's sense of wellbeing, his or her number of symptoms, and overall health. For example, Canadian researchers audiotaped more than 300 office visits with 39 different primary-care doctors. Patients were asked to rate the visit in terms of the relationship with their doctors. Then the researchers looked at how the patients' health fared over time. When patients reported that their doctors focused on their feelings and worries and listened to them carefully, they not only felt better, but objective measures showed they had fewer symptoms of disease.[22]

HONESTY & INTEGRITY

The development and recognition of these two key qualities takes time and trust. It is essential for patients to feel comfortable communicating openly how they really feel, often revealing deep, painful and personal aspects of their lives. Patients need to know that they will not be judged for sharing personal and family information, no matter what it is. A patient is equally responsible for instilling a sense of their own honesty and integrity in the DPR, since your doctor needs to know the truth about what's going on with your health condition in order to make informed observations and determinations about treatment.

Some patients want the doctor to be very direct about their condition and treatment, while other patients don't want to know too much; some go from the doctor-to-doctor looking for what they want to hear. It's a challenge when telling patients that they might not be cured or they will die. With integrity-based communications at the outset of the DPR, both doctor and patient understand the intentions and goals of each other, and proceed with mutual respect and confidence. Overall, most people want to share their stories and be part of the deeper interchange of information; they want to be heard. The people that I see want me to know about them and have me share what I see.

I DON'T KNOW

Doctors may often feel insecure or inadequate saying, "I don't know" when asked difficult questions about their patients' health condition. This lack of forthrightness may lead, however, to doctors trying to protect themselves, or to conceal their lack of knowledge by giving patients misinformation, inappropriate medications or guidance that are not in the patient's best interests. It can also lead to a doctor telling the patient that they need to learn to live with their condition or declaring their final predictions, such as "there's no hope for you, no treatment." It would be better to say simply, "I just don't know; maybe there is someone else who can help you."

An important quality for any health practitioner is "to know what you know and be aware and honest about what you don't know." When appropriate, be willing to admit any limitations in knowledge or experience that might affect a patient's health outcome. This involves a mixture of confidence, humility, care and compassion, and keeping education current with the latest information. The key is to keep the patient's best interests at heart. Yet, not all physicians think outside their own learned model. It helps to believe that there is a possibility for some miraculous or at least incremental change, which allows some hope even with a worst-case scenario.

TRUST & CONFIDENTIALITY

These qualities are necessary part of the DPR. Many patients may feel threatened by the relationship with their healthcare providers, due in part to previous experiences or a lack of education. Physicians at times feel pressured by patients' needs and demands—some of which may be unrealistic, unnecessary, or possibly even detrimental along with the required documentation and follow-up that many patients need. A good staff and support system is very helpful to streamline procedures and documentation, and facilitate efficiencies allowing for a quality experience between the Doctor and each Patient.

Trust provides comfort to patients. When we are ill or have been injured, it is comforting to turn to someone we trust, who we know cares about us (even though we may pay them and they don't come home with us). As children in our modern culture, this is typically the parents; as adults, we often seek either our doctor, a close member of our family or a dear friend depending upon the need and circumstances. Where matters involve spiritual issues we may turn to a respected and trusted minister, counselor or guide, or perhaps the world of nature.

Trust takes time and develops when we make wise decisions with our doctors from the start. We may find a doctor through our insurance company and begin a relationship, or we may be referred by a friend who believes in a particular doctor, and their trust gives us initial confidence. Yet, often, based on past experiences, we may not be someone who trusts easily, especially doctors, who become privy to our histories and our physical and psycho-emotional issues. With time and with testing the relationship and experiences, a bond can grow. Yet, most people cannot just trust blindly; they need to develop that over time.

"I trust you to be who you are, not what I wish you to be. It takes the investment of time and focus to achieve and nurture trust."

—ARGISLE

A healthy skepticism is also of value so individuals can make wise decisions about their path and care. Respect, or a sense of appreciation for the DPR, also allows good interaction whereas defensiveness and reactivity can block or worsen any good communication. Choosing wisely is part of the healing process.

A Good Patient – is aware of, honors and embraces the sacredness (centuries old) for this precious human healing relationship and the bond of doctor and patient. After all, you are seeking the best practitioner to help you heal and be healthy. Thus, make sure that you understand the doctor's perspective about treatment and healing and know as much about your prospective doctor as possible. That's your job as a good patient; trust is not one-sided.

Confidentiality is expected and needs to be an essential part of the entire medical profession, to be respected by the practitioners and entire staff. Now, there are a wide range of rules and laws that govern patient confidentiality, such as the HIPPA guidelines (Health Insurance Portability and Accountability Act, 1996) that clarify how medical information is handled. With many practices and hospitals converting to electronic records, patient privacy is even more highlighted. As we learn more about computer security, patient identity protection and confidentiality are now a concern for all of us.

Still, the basics of confidentiality go back to the essence of the DPR—**what a patient tells the doctor is private and not to be shared with anyone else.** This is especially true for the psychological fields of care, yet applies to all medical information. The doctor's staff must abide by this as well, and should not be talking about any specific patients other than in privacy with the practitioners and/or staff involved, and clearly not share any specifics with anyone outside the office.

THE OPPORTUNITY TO LEARN— EDUCATION IS A PRIORITY

Education is at the heart of any re-invention of our healthcare model. Discovering what factors in our lifestyle make a difference to our long-term health, such as avoiding smoking, getting adequate exercise, managing stress and eating plenty of fresh fruits and vegetables, we can educate wisely. Let's continue to educate teachers, healthcare providers, corporate participants and policy makers, as well as health practitioners and their staff—all to better educate patients, following the calling of "doctor as teacher." Our responsibility as individuals and healthcare consumers is to learn the basic principles of preventive care.

Look for a practice that offers the opportunity to learn more about Staying Healthy, and not just treating symptoms and diseases. This could be through the relationship with your physician and their staff as

> Education is an essential part of health improvement—knowing what to do to correct problems at their causative levels and making appropriate changes in behavior will influence better health outcomes.

well as through classes. Also, look for local talks and classes through colleges, natural food stores, pharmacies and hospitals, plus online information. For instance, Kaiser Permanente offers their millions of members numerous classes for improving health and lifestyle management (stress reduction, dealing with heart disease, diabetes, etc.)

Essential health education ideally begins with early learning in schools so that as children grow up they know and have the tools for life-long health. If we as patients can do our part, then our efforts will bear fruit and we can harvest our health as we age.

Prevention education is especially important for younger individuals (under 30 years old) who often think they are immortal because their bodies can tolerate considerable abuse in their early years. By the time these individuals reach their 30's and 40's, the consequences of such abuse however, may begin to manifest with enormous economic consequences for both individuals and society. This may be from high blood pressure or elevated cholesterol, blood sugar imbalance, which could precede diabetes, or the beginning of arthritis and even the development of cancer, which is often based on lifestyle habits. Since the vast majority of medical care and expenses occur in the oldest segment of our society (60+ years), this trend in costs escalates dramatically in the absence of early education and prevention.

Ideal Educational Goals:

- Provide education about the long-term, life-long benefits of preventive care which comes from positive self care and lifestyle;

- Reward behavior that fosters such preventive care with lower insurance rates for example, or rebates from employers for positive behaviors such as losing weight or stopping smoking;

- Discourage behavior and lifestyles that promote poor health in a variety of ways, with costly disincentives from insurances and employers as well as properly taxing food so that unhealthy choices and treats cost a bit more, as we have done nationally for cigarettes.

- Encourage a connection to nature's provisions and healing powers.

- Offer the best possible care to achieve the best outcomes.

Preferably, health education begins with families and their habits supported by parental guidance. Fortunately, many schools and government initiatives, like Michelle Obama's *Let's Move Program*, are focusing on the young with the educational guidelines for our public schools, with health classes and physical fitness.

WHAT'S ALREADY IN PLACE?

National guidelines have been developed for health curriculum development and promoting healthy environments at the schools; this includes wellness education, school meals and physical activity. In 2010, the CDC (Centers for Disease Control) published guidelines for schools to promote lifelong healthy eating.[23] They also developed model local school wellness policies aimed at preventing chronic illnesses. This policy monitors the quality of food offered at the school, and many schools since have eliminated sugar drinks and sodas with some changing vendors towards more organic and fresh foods.[24] School gardens and learning about labels and food ingredients are some good educational projects for young people.

However, it is only the states that put educational policies into action.[25] While the area of health education in the schools is mandated by each state, many states don't have any. Many existing programs are geared towards teaching about safe sex practices and avoiding alcohol while some states offer no required courses in health education. A national program funded by NIH (National Institute of Health) would go far in educating and motivating our youth to healthier positive behaviors.

For instance, California Project Lean[26] offers training and resources in English and Spanish to improve school meals and snacks, along with student exercise activities. Some states are setting environmental policies about pesticide use and air quality in the school. Today there are many healthy living issues besides diet and exercise that need to be addressed in our schools; these include general safety, guns and other weapons, and bullying. Time is an issue however: it's a crowded curriculum hungry for hours in the classroom, just as the doctor's office is often crowded with people waiting to be seen.

Also, many states have initiated school garden programs to teach children where their food comes from, how to grow it, and even how to prepare or cook it.[27] The Edible Schoolyard (ESY) project initiated twenty years ago in Berkeley, CA by the renowned chef Alice Waters has grown into a very successful nationwide program that now serves as a network and resource for schools throughout the US in building such programs.[28] There are currently over 4,000 programs across North America that are part of the ESY garden classrooms, school lunch programs, etc. ESY also gave birth to the National Farm-to-School network that brings local, often organic, food to the schools.[29] The federal Farm Bill of 2014 included a pilot project for procurement of unprocessed fruits and vegetables, and other federal programs to support farm to school programs have been funded. So even though there are impressive grass roots efforts to improve our youth's health, policy makers and educators need to find the time in the curriculum and funds in their already stretched budgets to initiate more programs. While the situation is improving, corporate sales of lower quality foods, like sweet sodas and candies, are still too commonplace in our schools. There needs to be more money raised to support healthier programs.

Special interest groups, who want their products promoted, whether it's the dairy and meat industries, soda manufacturers or others, should not sponsor age-appropriate educational materials. Even teachers and doctors should not be biased and provide the best health information that the government and schools can access.

What We Need to Know

By the time we graduate from high school, each of us should know how to answer the following questions.

- What are the needs for a healthy functioning human?

- What does it take to Stay Healthy for Life? (Long-range goals)

- What can I do to assure my own health, especially in the 5 key areas of Nutrition, Exercise, Stress, Sleep and Attitude?

- What health challenges do I face and how can I address them?

- How can I stay motivated to maintain healthy habits and avoid unhealthy ones?

- How healthy is my family and do I know their disease patterns?

- What family issues might challenge my health?

To help achieve these goals, I propose a variety of incentives be provided to individuals and educational institutions to promote awareness and education about preventive health. These include:

- *Educational grants and tuition support to promote broad-based learning of health principles to students at all levels of education.*

- *Discounted health insurance premiums for those who practice definitive preventive care and healthy lifestyles - how to evaluate and monitor needs to be developed and clarified.*

- *Tax breaks and other such financial inducements to individuals and companies that foster and nurture a culture of preventive health care, as well as tax consequences to companies for products sold that we know undermine health.*

Another important issue in health education is **health literacy**. This basically means how what is taught in schools gets carried to the parents as well as questioning the lack of understanding by heath consumers about the concept of risk and risk factors.[30] Health literacy affects a person's ability to navigate the healthcare system, communicate with their health providers, and engage in any self-care or chronic disease management. It's estimated that most adults in the US lack the skills needed to manage their health and prevent disease.[31]

OUR CHILDREN'S HEALTH IS OUR NATION'S FUTURE

Children's health and childhood obesity are worldwide issues that I have been talking and writing about for decades. The genesis of my interest in the health of children was my own childhood, when I needed to overcome my own weight issues, based on eating and overeating the new, industrialized American diet. What I have come to realize over the years is that we need a complete re-education for our families and children, with the support of our local, state and federal governments and our school system to instill in children both the awareness and incentives to create better food choices and eating habits. This is going to be a continual challenge in view of the multi-billion-dollar processed and fast food industries, the giant sugar soda conglomerates, and mega agriculture. To accomplish such change in our children's health outcomes will require a consistent and concerted effort from many sectors of society. One contribution I have made to this initiative was to create a kids' health education company, called Seasons Studios, with my creative colleague, Bethany Argisle. You can learn more at www.seasonsstudios.com.

Luckily, most of us as youngsters are blessed with fairly good health; yet over time we may undermine it with our improper self-care. For those of us who are adults, re-learning what it takes to support a healthy human body is key. It's never too late to change and when we do, even in later years, it can make a big difference in terms of how we feel and our level of health. I see this all the time in my Detox Groups when people experience the difference it makes in their wellbeing when they change their lifestyle and then make long-term decisions to stay with the changes.

SELF CARE

By educating our youth and by parents and teachers having good health information, we can begin to transform our culture from a "fix me" orientation to one based upon self-empowerment and responsibility—this is the true foundation for reforming our own health and our healthcare system. This will also benefit the health of our environment and the entire planet.

EXAMPLES OF HEALTH EDUCATIONAL PROGRAMS

BASIC PROGRAMS:
Many exist in the community, at clinics, or at schools

Lifestyle Assessment and Enhancement:
- Stress management
- Nutrition and eating habits—learning how to cook and what constitutes healthy meals and diet
- Exercise and body awareness
- Communication skills—learn how to get along with others easily

Behavior Modification for:
- Stopping smoking • Losing weight • Alcohol abuse

Healthy Aging
- Learn about essential risk factors that interfere with long-range health
- Look at any relevant testing to assess your health along the way; these may include breast checks and Pap tests in women, prostate checkups for men, and colonoscopies for appropriate people

Detox Practices
- Taking a week or month break from substances like sugar, caffeine, alcohol, etc. Also following an allergy elimination diet or alkaline-based diet to see how this helps with any health conditions
- Doing these activities in a group can help with motivation and follow through.

HEALTH CONDITION PROGRAMS:
- **General Health Support** for the "worried" well with no specific chronic condition—people who are basically healthy, but believe they are not. This involves general education about lifestyle choices and other aspects of healthy living.

Heart Disease
- Lessening risk factors – high blood pressure, cholesterol, stress

Cancer
- Preventive measures and contributory lifestyle factors
- Dealing with treatment, coping strategies for healing emotions and spirit, and support groups

OTHER DISEASES TO ADDRESS INCLUDE:
- Diabetes, Autoimmune diseases, AIDS, chronic pain.

THE AFFORDABILITY OF CARE

For most people the cost of medical care and how it will (or will not) be paid for is often the very first thing they consider. Thus, a key area of patient responsibility is to understand the basic financial relationship with their doctors and medical practices, including insurance coverage and any cost liabilities, plus the rules and the guidelines of each practice and practitioner. A lack of clarity here can lead to unfulfilled expectations in regard to services and/or unexpected costs, any of which can undermine the DPR and create stress.

Therefore, it is essential for patient and doctor to review the affordability of care. This typically involves a discussion of treatment options after the doctor has had an opportunity to assess the patient's health condition and consider possible approaches to treatment. Of course, there can be a wide variety of options, not all of which will be covered by insurance plans. By discussing the financial aspects and affordability of a plan between doctor (or staff member) and patient, both are assured that their agreed-to plan offers the best value, lowest risk, and most affordable overall option for the patient. In my own practice over the years, we have employed this proactive approach to discussing affordability of care with patients and have thus avoided many misunderstandings and disputes.

Of course, as with many areas including health care, it is the more affluent and educated individual that has a wider range of choices; thus, if you have money that you are willing to spend, you can see whom you wish and buy more services. What about those who can only afford what insurance or the government will cover? Currently they can get Western medicine approaches, but integrative and natural care or acupuncture is less available or even unavailable. That's why policies that proactively support health and prevention need to be adopted. With more dietary programs, natural remedies, and stress management supported by Medicare, for example, this would encourage insurance companies to follow suit.

As of 2012, about 33% of US adults have used complementary health practices, which include everything from yoga, meditation, supplements to utilizing complementary practitioners such as acupuncturists and massage therapists.[32] A recent survey[33] of 18 major HMOs and insurance providers, including Aetna, Medicare, Prudential, and Kaiser Permanente, found that 14 of them covered at least 11 of 34 complementary therapies; however, how much is covered and for which condition, varied considerably. Chiropractic, massage therapy and acupuncture are the three most-covered therapies followed by naturopathic medicine. Other therapies that are increasingly being included are herbal remedies, homeopathy, mind body stress management and meditation, but the extent of coverage is still quite limited.

Currently Medicare does not cover Alternative Medicine, such as homeopathy, naturopathy, acupuncture, holistic therapies and herbal medicine. In addition, Medicare does not cover Complementary Medicine, which often incorporates the use of spiritual, metaphysical and newly invented approaches to healing, as well as pre-modern medical practices.

Clearly, different people choose different avenues of care and treatment modalities based upon their budget, experiences, knowledge and belief systems. However, financially there is still not an equal playing field since most insurance plans mainly cover the Western model of medicine, requiring that almost all Natural and Eastern Medicine treatments be paid for out-of-pocket by the patient. Even in countries such as Canada and the U.K. that have a more socialized model of health care, what is covered is still primarily the Western approach. Fortunately, the situation is evolving, with increasing acceptance of integrative medicine mainstream programs; yet, there is still a long way to go.

CONCLUSION

A healthy relationship between doctor, or any healthcare provider, and patient is the cornerstone of true healing. The optimal DPR is a mutual relationship based on cooperation and communication. Care and compassion go heart in hand. If doctors are stressed and overwhelmed with demands and busyness, or if they are not healthy themselves, they cannot easily be fully present with their patients. Presence is so vital, and is at the heart of the DPR. Likewise a patients' punctuality and presence show respect to their healthcare provider and staff; as does being prepared with all necessary paperwork and questions.

Doctors need to be aware of how their practice schedules patients so as to not keep them waiting too long. Respect is also based on all the office interactions, not only with the physician but also with the medical, administrative and billing staff. It begins with the way the front desk staff treat patients, from the very first contact—by phone and in person—to the way appointments are made and how the subsequent business and billing transactions are handled, be they cash or with insurance.

How well are basic communications provided, such as returned phone calls, answers to questions, review of test results and follow-up appointments? From the perspective of the doctors' practices, it really helps when the patients share responsibility for these follow-ups and for supporting the practice so that most of the needs and actions, such as prescriptions, are completed during office visits. These elements combine to create and sustain a basic trust and comfort that allow patients and providers to have a positive healing experience.

Assess your DPR

Let's review where you are so far in your relationship with your primary physician. Rate on a 1–10 scale. from poor to excellent, how you feel about each topic we have discussed in this chapter. You might also re-prioritize the list based on what is most important for you. Also, feel free to add your own areas of concern.

- Shared Beliefs
- Compassion
- Being Present
- Mutual Respect
- Knowledge & Experience
- Confidence with Humility

- Personal Chemistry
- Honesty & Integrity
- Trust & Confidentiality
- The Opportunity to Learn
- Affordability

Now, what would you say about your DPR Evaluation?

- Are you happy and successful with your current doctor?
- Do you have a supportive, cooperative relationship with him or her?
- Can you ask questions or explain what alternative approaches you are using or considering?
- Do you have enough time at your appointment to discuss what you need?
- Do you feel heard?
- Are the staff at the office or clinic helpful and supportive?
- Is your family and/or primary relationship supportive?

Next, look at your responsibilities as a patient and rate yourself on how well you are doing, using the list below as a guide. This might include showing up on time for your appointments, making sure your insurance and/or payments are current with the office, and acknowledging the staff for the help they provide you.

Checklist for Being the Best Patient or Student of Health

- Know your rights – personal, medical and legal.
- Prepare ahead for your visit with your questions written and needs clarified.
- Communicate your needs clearly so that they can be addressed during your visit.
- Be responsible for understanding the business side of your relationship with your doctor and practice.
- Learn about the office policies and expectations.
- Be ready to provide the expected information and payments.
- Be respectful of the doctor and staff.
- Be sensitive to their time; assume that everyone in the practice is busy and doing their best.
- Be honest and responsible.
- Be willing to adapt as your health and healing change, and adjust over time.
- Trust in your own healing abilities.
- Expect and visualize healing (if that fits your belief system).
- Take responsibility for your health, and following through on the recommendations that you accept as correct for you.
- Stay Motivated!
- Let go of past negativity with other doctors or the healthcare system so that you can be present with your new doctor.
- Keep a positive attitude towards healing and others.

Health Bill of Rights for Patients

Ten ideas that empower each of us to embrace being recipients of optimal health care and help us to be discriminating in how we approach ourselves and our experiences within the healthcare system. Created by Elson Haas in collaboration with Bethany Argisle.

1. I have the right to make the final decision about what is done to my body.

2. I have the right to be treated with respect by my doctors and the staff in their offices and hospitals, and to have my needs respected.

3. I have the right to inquire about and to receive the best possible information and support about my condition.

4. I have the right to know the benefits and risks of any procedure or tests that I am asked to undertake, and expect support to make the right decisions.

5. I have the right to be informed about the expense for my treatment, tests or procedure, and to know what is covered or not covered by my insurance plan, and to challenge any undue expenses.

6. I have the right to explore and be told about any alternatives to the medically proposed treatments and the risks involved (both in the proposed treatments or alternatives), or to explore this with other experienced practitioners so that I can choose the best possible treatment.

7. I have the right to know and understand what my likely recovery will be for my condition or procedure (and associated costs), as well as the effects of not doing the prescribed treatment.

8. I have the right to be able to interview my doctors before and after any procedures or any proposed treatments (and be willing to pay for the doctor's time for such meetings). I would also like to be paid or provided some benefit in exchange for undue waiting times.

9. If in the hospital, I have the right to nourishing food and water, and am allowed to have my own food and nutritional supplements with me in respectful and appropriate collaboration with my medical treatment.

10. I have the right to bring in family members, (or other advocates) to help both with my decisions/choices about proposed treatments, and to see how they can be included in my recovery along with my active healthcare providers.

NOTE: See Doctor's Bill of Rights in Appendix 2

A PREVIEW

NEW MEDICINE SOLUTIONS

Integrating Natural, Eastern and Western
Approaches to Correct Common Medical Conditions

New Medicine Solutions is the healthy application of the ideas and principles found in this book to many common health problems. This next volume of *NEW Medicine* offers a simple understanding of the biology of each condition and provides integrated Natural, Eastern and Western treatment strategies. These safe and relatively simple approaches can lessen symptoms, ameliorate specific conditions, prevent or delay their progression, and improve overall health.

Many of these treatments have proven successful in multiple studies and with my patients over the years.

Table of Contents

CHAPTER SUMMARIES

CHAPTER 1 – Weight Management and Obesity

This chapter focuses on the more serious consequences of body weight and poor fitness that primarily result from unhealthy food choices and a sedentary lifestyle. How can we address these important issues? It is a known fact that general diet and nutrition—what we eat—influences the causes, prevention, and healing of virtually all the conditions described in this book. Our food choices also affect our basic health, energy, weight, mood, and likely what diseases we develop.

- Excess weight has become a national problem of epidemic proportions. In this chapter, I explore the political issues of food production and advertising, and the biological consequences of our daily choices. Why does too much weight put us at risk for illness and what approaches are considered the most useful in losing weight and keeping it off? I offer a practical overview of lifestyle choices for managing our eating habits and preventing long-term ill effects of being overweight.

- **Obesity** and the need for **Weight Management** are results of both our genetics and our life-long habits, often based on our family upbringing and diet. Our tendency to be overweight can also begin in utero (thus, pregnant moms need to pay attention too). Common periods in our lives for overeating and weight gain are during transitions and stressful times. Examples include adolescence and menopause with related changes in body hormones that play a part in weight management. How much our diet affects our disease patterns varies from problem to problem and person to person. That's why exploring our own food issues can offer great assistance in healing. **Typically, our nutritional habits must be challenged and often changed to make a difference in our long-term health.**

CHAPTER 2 – Diabetes, The Sugar/Carb Connection:
Consequences, Treatment and Prevention

Both types of diabetes are explored here with the focus on type 2 (usually adult onset), a growing concern because of its connection to being over-weight along with the modern day, processed food diet and lack of exercise. Types 1 and 2 can both lead to other medical conditions including cardiovas-cular disease, neuropathy (nerve pain and loss of function), kidney disease, and visual problems.

- **Diabetes is a concerning and expensive disease** with the economic costs to the individual, insurance, and the healthcare system in the trillions per year. This is a major problem that can be largely PREVENTED and definitely lessened, primarily through nutrition, fitness and weight management.

- **The key nutritional focus is to minimize refined flour and sugar products**—lowering CARBS— fewer baked goods, sweets, sodas for sure, and even fruit juices.

- It is also important to learn about the **Glycemic Index**—how quickly spe-cific foods get into our blood stream, increase our blood sugar levels, and influence pancreatic insulin release.

- **Some nutrients** that can be helpful in controlling blood sugar levels are chromium, glutamine, alpha lipoic acid, and cinnamon.

- **Fitness is the foundation and reducing body fat is the focus.**

CHAPTERS 3 & 4 – The Immune System:
Discussed together as two aspects of a similar issue

Chapter 3: Hypo Immunity and Infectious Diseases
Chapter 4: Hyper Immunity—Allergies and Autoimmune Diseases

This discussion begins with a simple summary of how the healthy immune system functions, what undermines immunity, and then provides strategies to help bring the immune system back into balance.

Immune responses are a natural function of our bodies that embrace many levels of life. The dynamic balance of the immune system is influenced by multiple factors—genetics and body constitution, nutrition, stress, mental attitudes, relationships, chemical and metal exposures, gastrointestinal function, as well as past medical conditions and their treatments. The use of immunosuppressive steroids and repeated courses of antibiotics can lay the ground for more long-term immune problems. Vaccines also cause immune interplay and may stress the body. The gut and the *microbiome* (our intestinal microbial environment) are being shown to influence immunity as much as any factor.

CHAPTER 3 discusses Immune Depression, or hypo-activity, which typically leads to us getting infections more easily, (especially from viruses and other microbes) whereas **Immune Hyper-reactivity, discussed in Chapter 4,** results in the ever-growing problems of allergies and autoimmune conditions, such as Rheumatoid Arthritis and Hashimoto's Thyroiditis.

I see that more frequent infections occur when the body "terrain" (our tissue state) is imbalanced—weakened, stressed, congested, or overly acidic. This creates a better host for various microbes, which can overpower our immune warriors and cause trouble. To make a difference, we must assess where we are in terms of nutritional status (deficiency and toxicity), hidden microbial problems, and various stressors, and then restore better lifestyle habits, such as improved diet and proper sleep. Of course, overwhelming microbial invasion causes problems in the healthiest body. Still, maintaining our health is the only sensible way to prevent infections. At the same time healthy immunity helps us to recover more readily when we do get sick.

CHAPTER 4 – Hyperactivity of the immune system is currently a more significant and common problem in the US than low immunity, with allergies, autoimmune diseases and asthma on the increase. I explore the biology of these conditions as well as strategies to prevent them from developing in the first place or treating them with NEW Medicine approaches when needed.

For a detailed discussion of this topic see my recent book, *Ultimate Immunity,* co-authored with Dr. Sondra Barrett and published by Rodale Books (2014).

CHAPTER 5 – Mood and Energy Disorders:
Fatigue, Insomnia, Depression, and Anxiety

This chapter begins by defining what energy is and how it affects our moods, sleep, and wellbeing. What is the role of stress on energy depletion and what steps can we take to become more aware to lessen the drain on our life force? We offer questions to help you evaluate your energy level and management as well as solutions to improve your health.

- Too much (hyper) or imbalanced energy can cause **anxiety** and **insomnia** while too little or weak energy (hypo) may bring **fatigue** and **depression.** Also, there's a relationship and interaction between all of these states— they cross over each other like four rings linked together—insomnia affects fatigue and energy levels, while anxiety and depression can feed on each other. These are all various aspects of the complex hyper-hypo energy continuum, ranging from low energy to extreme agitation.

- **First, assess your lifestyle habits** to see where energy imbalances come from. This may be from caffeine, sugar and drug use, plus previous illnesses and their treatments, exercise activities, sleep patterns and stress issues, as well as your age and developmental stage of life. Get to know your needs and change with them consistently. Monitor and minimize stimulating and sedating substances that are so commonly used to alter or control our energies. Of course, substance abuse at any age is problematic.

• **Fatigue, Insomnia, Anxiety, and Depression** are so common in our modern/techno-cultures and many people being out of sync with their natural cycles—with excess work and life schedules that are anti-nature and seasonally imbalanced, such as having too many demands in the winter and at holiday times. How do we address these without changing our life focus?

• **All of these issues are more common as we age** and hormones change. We should examine thyroid and adrenal hormone function as well as sex hormones and brain neurotransmitters as there are many common symptoms that point to poor function in these key areas. Exposure to electromagnetic frequencies can also affect our moods and energy.

• **Therapies** discussed include diet and natural supplements, exercise (outer and inner), mind-body healing, natural (bio-identical) hormone balancing, and acupuncture and herbal therapies.

CHAPTER 6 – Healthy Aging

• **We are currently living longer than our ancestors**, and facing new challenges due to the reduction, or loss of hormones, lowered muscle mass, bone loss, and worsening memory. The role that various life issues play in healthy aging is reviewed, with ways to stay healthier longer by being more active and vital as a result of positive lifestyle choices.

• **Memory and brain functions are crucial** and can be challenging as we age. I present many NEW Medicine approaches to support a healthy, functioning brain.

- **Cardiovascular and bone health** are central to staying youthful and fit. **Heart and Vascular problems** are still the number one cause of a shortened life span.

- **NEW Medicine** approaches to maintain our health and vitality are keys and here the Natural and Eastern therapies are a very helpful adjunct to Western practice. Staying in tune with the seasons of the year and of our lives is a good way to stay attuned to our best health—this is the basis of my first book, *Staying Healthy with the Seasons*.

CHAPTER 7 – Hormones and Health

Hormones play a vital role in healthy aging and many other medical issues. Here, we address all of the active hormones that regulate the body, especially thyroid and adrenal functions, plus pancreas and sugar metabolism. Then, we look at those hormones that change (lower) as we age and the safety of bio-identical (versus synthetic) hormone replacement—and remind you that sexual health, cholesterol, and hormones are linked together.

- **Measuring hormone levels**—thyroid, adrenal, estrogen, progesterone, testosterone and DHEA—helps to track the body state. These hormones play a part in hundreds of functions daily, many of them in the brain and nervous system. Thus, supporting them with bio-identical hormones (having the same chemical structure that your body produces) often helps many people continue to feel youthful and age better. These programs are basically safe and useful without the risk levels of using synthetic hormones, yet more studies are still needed to confirm this.

- **Programs need to be individualized** and should be overseen by an experienced medical practitioner, Natural or Western, or even a nutritionist, although an MD or ND would be needed for prescription hormones.

CHAPTER 8 – Gastrointestinal (GI) Problems:
Irritable Bowel Syndrome, Parasites and Yeast Issues

Gastrointestinal health is crucial to overall wellbeing and in this chapter I cover how the healthy GI tract works, factors that contribute to GI problems, the best tests to evaluate them, plus ways to improve overall GI function.

- First, we assess the patient's complaints, diet and travel activities—all of which can challenge digestive function and overall health. Gastrointestinal health is mainly influenced by food choices and habits, as well as the effects of previous treatments with medicines, especially antibiotics.

- **I review tests used to evaluate the GI tract**—assessing gut function and microbial status. Are the right microbes present with no pathogenic or problematic bacteria, yeast or parasites? As with IBS (Irritable Bowel Syndrome), it is often foods and microbes that cause imbalance and symptoms, plus stress—all of which can lead to reduced enzymes and stomach acid, inflammation, and then the many symptoms resulting from these factors.

- **Use natural treatments and prescriptions** to eradicate problematic organisms and restore and help heal the gut lining and function—all part of the 5-R Program of Removal, Restoration, Re-innoculation, Repair, and Rebalance—described fully in my book, *The Detox Diet* (2012).

- **With problems like inflammation** (such as colitis), GI upset (like pain or bloating), or with Irritable Bowel Syndrome (IBS), we look at contributory factors, which are most commonly reactive foods, irritating microbes like amoebas, or *Blastocystis hominis*, and stress, since the GI tract is extremely sensitive to psycho-emotional factors. Restoring good anatomy—tissue health for proper function and assimilation—takes time and will benefit immune activity and aging.

CHAPTER 9 – Cardiovascular Disease

Cardiovascular disease is still the number one killer in the US, and this chapter covers the NEW Medicine understanding of contributory factors—mainly lifestyle choices. Solutions include a more vegetable-focused diet, regular exercise and weight reduction, stress management, and natural supplements. There are many options in medical care and, as always, we should look at the **risks versus the benefits** of any treatment.

- **WM definitely offers support here**, yet it is limited in the areas of prevention where diet, stress, emotions, and genetic predispositions are very important. WM therapies can be lifesaving for heart attacks or heart arrhythmias and in such cases most people generally consider WM interventions, yet these treatments can also be invasive and injurious and need extended recovery time. Here, reducing risks is the wise place to start and continue. Once problems occur, we want to repair whatever CVD damage is present.

- **Healthy Lifestyle has a bigger impact on Cardiovascular Health than Genetics,** and this is likely true for all chronic conditions. Our genes may predispose us towards certain diseases, yet our life choices cause them to play out, or not, in many cases. One study suggested the **five most important healthy behaviors are: not smoking, low or no alcohol intake, weight control, physical activity, and a healthy diet.**

- **Each individual case must be reviewed to create the best plan for both preventing and treating CVD.** Taking into account all possible causative factors and remedies is key to a helpful treatment program.

CHAPTER 10 – Cancer

As with all the chapters in *NEW Medicine Solutions*, we offer a biological overview—presenting current understanding of the cancer disease process. We discuss the role of genetics and epigenetics, including the effect of dietary choices, weight and other habits on the development of cancer. What role does the immune system play here, if any, and what can we do to help prevent the most personally frightening disease of our times? The current Western model of treatment is based on cytotoxic (cell toxicity) approaches like chemotherapy, which can also damage healthy cells. Our integrative NEW Medicine approach looks at supportive measures when, or if, a person gets cancer, as well as theories of prevention and its importance as the most sensible approach to cancer.

- As with CVD, diet, stress and other lifestyle issues are closely aligned with a higher risk of developing many cancers—scientists often state that up to 70% of such risk is attributable to our lifestyle.

- **Individualized care** is especially important with cancer therapies so it is important to assess risks versus benefits when choosing the right treatment plan. I review some of the important points of common cancers like Breast, Prostate, Colon, and Lung. Nowadays people often combine Western treatments and other alternative, nutritional, and mind/body therapies.

CHAPTER 11 – Chronic Pain Conditions:
Back and Neck, Arthritis, Headaches, and Skin Conditions

Chronic debilitating pain is a distressing issue for people and their physicians, and a common reason for visiting the doctor. Quality of life is affected, and having persistent pain can result in other emotional and psychological problems, with the effects of drug use and related dependency issues. The causes (typically injuries and inflammation) of different kinds of pain are varied and find expression in many forms, mainly low back pain, neck pain and headaches, and joint pains. Additional challenges come from the meaning an individual gives to pain and the psycho-emotional stress that can arise. Does the pain mean a disease is worsening? Is the pain related to stress? Are there structural imbalances? Can we find viable solutions or even prevent the pain from getting worse? These are all important questions and NEW Medicine approaches can often offer helpful solutions.

- **Back pain** is likely the most common disabling pain, especially of the low back and neck. Injuries can be a common cause. Of course, the effects of wear and tear, as in osteoarthritis, can produce significant and persistent pain. Headaches can be troubling as well and I discuss the many factors that may contribute to them plus NEW therapeutic approaches.

- NEW Medicine Treatments to help reduce inflammation and pain can include nutritional and detoxification programs, natural and herbal remedies, acupuncture, and structural corrective therapies.

- **Skin Conditions** are also quite common and often a result of body reactions and toxicity. As in most WM treatments that use an "outside-in" approach, we often apply creams to rashes, be they allergies, or from unknown causes, yet I like to suggest, "We heal the skin from 'inside out' rather than solely approaching from the outside treatment."

APPENDIX 1

CHRONIC DISEASE IN THE US

Let's look more closely at the high incidence and costliness/expense of three of our major Chronic Diseases – **Cardiovascular Disease, Cancer and Diabetes.**

- As of 2015, about half of all adults had one or more chronic health conditions.[1]

- It's estimated that about 70% of all deaths in the US are due to chronic illness.[2]

- Treating chronic diseases accounts for nearly 86% of annual US health care expenditures.[3]

Improved diagnostics and treatments have lead to lower mortality rates, but the costs of managing chronic problems have risen. We are able to keep people living longer, yet does this really improve *health*? It can, of course, but do people have a better quality of life, or they just experience a longer, slower demise? A significant portion of healthcare costs accrue during the last few months of life, although this trend is beginning to change with more aware-ness regarding palliative care and health directives (people requesting less life-prolonging interventions). Medicare spending during the year of death for people over 70 has been decreasing, suggesting a change toward less intensive and costly end-of-life strategies.[4]

The Obesity Epidemic

We have been seeing a significant rise in the incidence of Obesity over recent decades, yet with some leveling off in the last few years. Obesity itself is not fatal, yet it does increase the risk of the key three life-threatening diseases mentioned above. In fact, some would argue that calling Obesity a disease is controversial[5] although in 2013 the AMA declared that it is.[6] Obesity greatly increases the probability of multiple life-threatening chronic problems, especially diabetes and also increases cancer and cardiovascular risks.

This trend is particularly alarming among young people because when these issues start earlier they will affect long-term health, with less chance for quality of life, plus the additional costs of treatment for each person (or their insurance company), possibly their family, and the entire healthcare system. The rising direct costs of treating chronic illnesses are just the tip of the iceberg; there is also an enormous cost to us individually and as a society in reduced quality of life, lost productivity and chronic illness's effects on family members.

The good news is that many chronic conditions and diseases can be prevented, delayed, or minimized by integrative health approaches and positive lifestyle changes.

FIVE BEHAVIORS THAT PUT OUR HEALTH AT RISK

- Lack of physical activity[7]
- Poor nutrition - eating few fresh fruits or vegetables[8]
- Unhealthy weight[9]
- Tobacco use[10]
- Excessive alcohol consumption[11]

In a study[12] of 2000 men lasting 30 years, those who addressed at least four of the above unhealthy behaviors had much lower incidence of chronic diseases—namely cancer, cardiovascular, diabetes, and cognitive decline.

Our challenge as a community of healthcare providers and patients is first to educate people about the benefits of preventive and integrative healthcare, then to empower and support one another to practice such healthcare in our daily lives.

Of course, there are other chronic problems such as arthritis, back pain, skin rashes and insomnia that contribute to significant suffering and pain, with considerable financial costs associated with treatment and work time lost. Many natural and NEW Medicine remedies may also work well for such conditions. These solutions can be even more effective when integrated into a comprehensive program of diet and lifestyle change, nutritional and herbal supplements, and if necessary, prescription medicines.

The treatment and prevention of worsening chronic problems are most effective when begun early. The key here is to identitfy underlying causes, which are strongly linked to lifestyle choices including diet, exercise, and improving stress management skills. An important part of the NEW Medicine approach is a particular understanding of the causes of disease that I have developed during my career, and which I discuss in detail in Chapter 3.

Michael M has been my patient since 1998. He worked and traveled a lot and was 30 pounds overweight and taking several medications for early diabetes along with high cholesterol and blood pressure, a common mixture for men in their 40's and 50's living the American Dream. It took work to get him motivated to eat differently and he was part of one of my detox groups. As he lost weight and used some natural remedies, he was able to get off all medicines and have control of his glucose, blood pressure and other numbers. Over the years, as he was more or less diligent with his lifestyle, he was also on and off medicines. He also experienced the benefits of feeling much better at many levels when he followed what we may call a "healthy lifestyle program."

CARDIOVASCULAR DISEASE (CVD)[13]

- It is estimated that more than 30% of the population have some form of CVD.
- It is the leading cause of death.
- *CVD problems can be managed and even lessened by lifestyle changes, specifically in the areas of diet, exercise and stress management.*

CANCER[14]

- Cancer is second leading cause of death—in 2015 cancer was estimated to have caused over 1,500 deaths each day.
- The lifetime risk of developing some form of cancer is 39.6%.[15]
- *Evidence suggests that about one-third of cancer deaths are related to overweight or obesity, physical inactivity and poor nutrition, and thus could be prevented.*
- *It is estimated that 30% of cancer deaths are caused by tobacco use and are thus preventable.*
- *Many skin cancers could also be prevented by protection from the sun's rays and avoiding indoor tanning.*

DIABETES[16]

- An estimated 29 million Americans currently have Diabetes.
- The CDC projects that the number could grow to 1 in 5 or even 1 in 3 by mid-century.
- Diabetes is the 7th leading cause of death in the US.
- 25% of diabetes cases are undiagnosed.
- People with Diabetes have a 2–4 times greater risk for heart disease deaths and stroke.
- Diabetes is a leading cause of complications such as blindness, kidney failure and lower extremity amputations.

- In 2012, the combined costs for Diabetes care totaled 1 in every 5 healthcare dollars spent—more than expenditures for AIDS and all cancers combined.
- ***Most Diabetes is preventable.*** *Type 2 Diabetes, the most common form, develops primarily from lifestyle issues like diet, overweight and lack of exercise.*

THE OBESITY EPIDEMIC[17, 18]

- 34.9% of US adults are obese—up from 20% in 1991[19] and 15% in 1980.
- Approximately 17% (12.7 million) of children and adolescents aged 2-19 years are obese; another 14% are overweight. (In 1980 both numbers were 6%).
- The good news is that obesity in children aged 2-5 years has decreased from 13.9% (2003-2004) to 8.4% (2011-12).
- More than 25% of all health care costs are related to obesity, over-weight and physical inactivity.
- Obesity-related conditions include heart disease, stroke, type 2 diabetes and certain types of cancer—some of the leading causes of preventable death.
- *Most obesity cases can be treated or prevented by lifestyle and behavior changes in the obvious areas of dietary choices and physical fitness.*

APPENDIX 2

THE DOCTOR'S SIDE OF THE DPR

Here's some more material on the Doctor-Patient Relationship that is more focused on physicians and what I would like my colleagues to think about. How close are you to some of these attributes? As doctors and practitioners we never stop learning and our experience with each patient is as unique for us as it is for her or him.

Being the Best Doctor

- Take care of yourself; when you are healthy, you can be the best healer.

- Keep knowledge current and be willing to say, "I don't know."

- Learn about new tests and treatments.

- Enjoy what you do.

- Show care and compassion.

- Be respectful of patients' views even if you disagree.

- Be a good listener—be present.

- Be on time and honor your patient's time.

- Be open-minded or tolerant of your patient's beliefs.

- Look for causes and order appropriate tests.

- Support health, even beyond money factors.

- Create a healthy work environment.

- Be kind and considerate to your staff.

- Review regularly your administrative and medical staff and your policies.

- Exude confidence with humility in your work.

- Stay positive, or at least balanced, in your assessments.

- Know that your words have power to enhance or diminish healing, or cause stress; be cautious about what you say and how you say it.

Education and Communication for Staff and Patients

Healthcare practitioners and their practices may begin re-inventing ways that promote preventive care and a truly meaningful relationship between Doctors, (and staff) and their Patients. Education needs to include medical staff as well. Some of the ways to accomplish these goals are with the following suggestions:

• Staff Education—The doctors, nurses, and other healthcare practitioners are ideally well educated and informed to deliver the best possible medical care. It is also imperative that the administrative and support staff be educated and informed about how to relate and communicate with their patients, in order to deliver the highest quality supportive care . In this way patients will feel they are being treated with dignity and respect, and the typical interpersonal stresses associated with the healthcare experience may be minimized.

• Communication & Teamwork—Fostering communication and teamwork between practitioners and staff is essential in making a difference in patient care, office morale and working together as a healthcare team. This helps to support the patients with the best possible care. Working in a medical setting is a service that requires compassion and connection; thus staff members who don't feel well enough or emotionally strong enough to give of themselves are not likely the best ones for the job. At the outset,it helps to let all employees and staff know what expectations you have for their work.

In my practice, we facilitate communication between staff and providers through a variety of strategies, which allows for a greater connectedness and commitment to doing the best job. Some of these include:

- Periodic staff meetings, where concerns and solutions are addressed

- Offsite events for families of the practice such as picnics and dinners, a boat ride and related local activities

- In-house newsletters

- Profit Sharing and Bonuses, which raises morale and supports the team spirit.

Doctor's Bill of Rights

In addition to the Patient Bill of Rights at the end of Chapter 4, here are some healthy guidelines for physicians. Since completing medical school in Ann Arbor, Michigan back in the early 1970s, my focus has been patient care. Yet, to have a good working doctor—patient relationship we need mutual collaboration and respect to achieve each person's ideal health outcome.

This Doctors' Bill of Rights emerged after many years of daily clinical experience with patients and with my healthcare colleagues.

1. Doctors have the right to be human, and at times—despite their best efforts—they may make mistakes. Thus, doctors have a right to be wrong. In this way they don't need to practice such defensive medicine and order so many tests when they believe the patient does not have a specific problem, for example doing a head x-ray or CAT Scan on every child with a head trauma. "Wait and see" becomes more acceptable.

2. Doctors have the right to say, "I don't know" and should say so when they really don't know the diagnosis or best treatment plan. They can then consult with their colleagues before making the final determination about a patient's condition and treatment plan. They

will not know everything; no one does. Each doctor should maintain a referral list of local practitioners that they trust.

3. Doctors have the right to charge people for their time (especially in fee-for-service practices) as well as when patients need special care, and bill appropriately for their services. Whether they charge for research or consultation with other practitioners should be discussed with each patient or given as a practice policy.

4. Doctors and their practices have the right to set up criteria, guidelines, and boundaries for accepting and working with their patients.

5. Doctors have the right to ask patients for the information they need to care for them, and request that patients fill out their forms honestly.

6. Doctors and patients should practice honesty with one another, and physicians have the right to select the patients they can work and cooperate best with to provide the appropriate treatments.

7. Doctors have the right to inform patients when they no longer feel they can help—for whatever reason— in their healing and/or recovery, and if not, they can refer them to another physician.

8. Doctors have the right to select the kinds of treatments they believe in and practice, and it's up to the patients to decide what treatment they wish to accept—all part of mutual cooperation.

9. Doctors have the right to dismiss patients if—after being notified—they are abusive to the physicians or staff, or if they refuse to compensate the practice for its services. As mentioned above, they can also refer patients to other practitioners if they don't feel they can help them.

10. Doctors have the right to set up the practice model they choose, and decide if it is in true healthful service and supports their desires and beliefs about their work.

REFERENCES

INTRODUCTION REFERENCES

1 http://data.worldbank.org/indicator/SH.XPD.TOTL.ZS

2 The Healthiest (and Least Healthy) Countries in the World - 24/7 Wall St. http://247wallst. com/special-report/2015/04/03/the-healthiest-and-least-healthy-countries-in-the-world/#ixz-z3owY5rbkL

3 http://www.cbsnews.com/news/u-s-health-care-system-ranks-lowest-in-international-survey/

4 http://www.usatoday.com/story/money/2015/04/03/24-7-wall-st-healthiest-countries/70859728/

5 PwC: Healthcare Spending Growth Rate to Dip 6.5% in 2016 by Staff Writer 06/10/2015 0 Comments http://hitconsultant.net/2015/06/10/pwchealthcare-spending-growth-rate-to-dip/

6 http://www.healthbeatblog.com/2009/08/who-is-making-the-biggest-profits-from-us-health-care-you-might-be-surprised-.html.

7 AMERICA'S BITTER PILL Money, Politics, Backroom Deals, and the Fight to Fix Our Broken Healthcare System By Steven Brill Random House

8 Bitter Pill: Why Medical Bills are Killing US. Time April 4, 2013. http://time.com/198/bitter-pill-why-medical-bills-are-killing-us/

9 http://www.cdc.gov/nchs/fastats/drug-use-therapeutic.htm

10 http://www.theatlantic.com/business/archive/2013/03/why-is-american-health-care-so-ridic-ulously-expensive/274425/

11 http://www.theatlantic.com/business/archive/2013/03/why-is-american-health-care-so-ridiculously-expensive/274425/

12 http://e360.yale.edu/feature/as_pharmaceutical_use_soars_drugs_taint_water_and_wild-life/2263/015.pdf

13 http://prescriptiondrugs.procon.org/#background

14 http://www.cdc.gov/biomonitoring/pdf/FourthReport_UpdatedTables_Feb2015.pdf

15 Globally the US medical device companies have generated revenues that exceed $110 billion. (2012) see select http://selectusa.commerce.gov/industry-snapshots/medical-de-vice-industry-united-states. SB

16 PWC. Medical cost trend: Behind the numbers. 2016.http://www.pwc.com/us/en/health-industries/behind-the-numbers/behind-the-numbers-2016.html

17 America's epidemic of unnecessary care – Atul Gawande http://www.newyorker.com/magazine/2015/05/11/overkill-atul-gawande

18 Reid, TR. The Healing of America: A Global Quest for Better, Cheaper, and Fairer Health Care. Penguin Books 2010

19 http://www.jacksonhealthcare.com/media-room/news/gallup-release-v2/

20 Geyman, J. The Decline of Primary Care: http://pnhp.org/blog/2011/08/09/the-decline-of-primary-care-the-silent-crisis-undermining-u-s-health-care/

CHAPTER 1 REFERENCES

1   "The Operator" by Michael Specter. The New Yorker, February 4, 2013

2   http://consumer.healthday.com/encyclopedia/high_blood_pressure_24/blood_pressure_news_70/salt_and_hypertension_645421.html

3   Bioidentical hormones: help or hype. Harvard Health Publications 2011. http://www.health.harvard.edu/womens_health/bioidentical_hormones_help_or_hype

4   https://www.nlm.nih.gov/medlineplus/herbalmedicine.html

5   The American Botanical Council _ http://abc.herbalgram.org

6   http://www.anmcb.org/certificationinformation.html

7   http://www.chopra.com/our_services/ayurveda

8   Origins of Chinese Medicine www.drshen.com/chineseherbsorigin.html _

9   http://umm.edu/health/medical/altmed/treatment/acupuncture

10 Kaptchuk Ted. The Web That Has No Weaver: Understanding Chinese Medicine. 2nd Edition. McGraw_Hill, 2000

11 Beinfeld H and E Korngold. Between Heaven and Earth: A Guide to Chinese Medicine. Ballentine Books, 1992.

12 [http://www.takingcharge.csh.umn.edu/explore_healing_practices/traditional_chinese_medicine/what_qi_and_other_concepts)

13 http://nccam.nih.gov/news/press/12172014

14 Vickers AJ, Cronin AM, Maschino AC, et al. Acupuncture for chronic pain: individual patient data meta_analysis. *Archives of Internal Medicine*. September 10, 2012; Epub ahead of print.

15 Han JS. Acupuncture and endorphins. Neurosci Lett. 2004 May 6;361(1_3):258_61

16 http://www.biosonics.com/About_Our_Site.html

17 http://www.credentialingexcellence.org/p/cm/ld/fid=86

18 http://nccam.nih.gov/health/cancer/camcancer.htm#use

19 http://www.fda.gov/NewsEvents/Newsroom/PressAnnouncements/2004/ucm108379.htm

20 Rabin, R.C. Burnt Out Primary Care Docs Are Voting With Their Feet. April 1, 2014. http://khn.org/news/doctor_burnout/

21 Sanghavia, D. The Phantom Menace of Sleep-Deprived Doctors. *The New York Times Magazine*, AUG. 5, 2011http://www.nytimes.com/2011/08/07/magazine/the-phantom-menace-of-sleep-deprived-doctors.html?_r=0

22 http://www.drweil.com/drw/u/QAA401226/Are-Saliva-Tests-Any-Good.html

23 Agency for Healthcare Research and Quality. Guideline Summary NGC-10090. Summary recommendations for clinical preventive services Nov. 2013.http://www.guideline.gov/content.aspx?id=47554&search=preventive+and+clinical+preventive+services

24 Andrew Weil. Spontaneous Healing : How to Discover and Embrace Your Body's Natural Ability to Maintain and Heal Itself Ballentine Books 2000

25 http://www.nhs.uk/Conditions/homeopathy/Pages/Introduction.aspx#available; http://www.publications.parliament.uk/pa/cm200910/cmselect/cmsctech/45/4504.htm#a5

26 Ullman, D. Homeopathic medicine: Europe's #1 Alternative for Doctors. http://www.huffingtonpost.com/dana-ullman/homeopathic-medicine-euro_b_402490.html

27 Bei-JHung Chang et al. Relaxation response and spirituality: Pathways to improve psychological outcomes in cardiac rehabilitation. J. Psychosomatic Research 69: 2: 93-100, 2010. DOI: http://dx.doi.org/10.1016/j.jpsychores.2010.01.007

CHAPTER 2 REFERENCES

1 Pelletier, Kenneth R. and Robert Lutz (1988) Healthy People — Healthy Business: A Critical Review of Stress Management Programs in the Workplace. *American Journal of Health Promotion: Winter 1988*, Vol. 2, No. 3, pp. 5-19.doi: http://dx.doi.org/10.4278/0890-1171-2.3.5

2 Willet, Walter et al. Prevention of Chronic Disease by Means of Diet and Lifestyle Changes. p 836-850.Chapter 44 in Disease Control Priorities in Developing Countries. 2nd edition. DT Jamieson et al editors. World Bank 2006

3 Ford, Earl S. et al. Healthy Living Is the Best Revenge: Findings From the European Prospective Investigation Into Cancer and Nutrition-Potsdam Study. *Arch Intern Med.*, 2009; 169 (15): 1355-1362

4 Kanaya, Alka M. et al. TheLive Well, Be Well Study: A Community-Based, Translational Lifestyle Program to Lower Diabetes Risk Factors in Ethnic Minority and Lower–Socioeconomic Status Adults. American Journal of Public Health, 2012; DOI: 10.2105/AJPH.2011.300456

5 http://www.nhlbi.nih.gov/health/health-topics/topics/hd/preven.

6 Anand, P. et al. Cancer is a Preventable Disease that Requires Major Lifestyle Changes. *Pharm Res.* 2008 Sep; 25(9): 2097–2116.Published online 2008 Jul 15. doi: 10.1007/s11095-008-9661-9

7 Kenneth R. Pelletier and Robert Lutz *(1988)* Healthy People — Healthy Business: A Critical Review of Stress Management Programs in the Workplace. American Journal of Health Promotion: Winter 1988, Vol. 2, No. 3, pp. 5-19.doi: http://dx.doi.org/10.4278/0890-1171-2.3.5

8   ToobertDJ et al. Biologic and Quality_of_Life Outcomes from the Mediterranean Lifestyle Program Diabetes Care 26:2288–2293, 2003

9   Sondra Barrett. Secrets of Your Cells: Discovering your body's inner intelligence. Sounds True Boulder, CO. 2013.

10 GL Wolff et al. Maternal epigenetics and methyl supplements affect agouti gene expression in A^{vy}/a mice. The FASEB Journal 12 (11): 949_957, 1998

11 Ornish, D. et al. Changes in prostate gene expression in men undergoing an intensive nutrition and lifestyle intervention. Proceedings of the National Academy of Sciences (PNAS) 105(24):8369_8374, 2008.

CHAPTER 3 REFERENCES

1   Lifestyle Medicine: Evidence Review for Lifestyle Interventions. American College of Preventive Medicine. June 30, 2009 https://www.acpm.org/resource/resmgr/lmi_files/lifestylemedicine_literature.pdf

2   http://gmo_awareness.com/shopping_list/smart_phone_apps/

3   http://appcrawlr.com/ios_apps/best_apps_food_labels

4   Read more at: http://www.azquotes.com/quote/811343

5   Selye H. The Stress of Life. New York: McGraw-Hill; 1956. Selye H. The physiology and pathology of exposure to stress. Acta;1975.

6   http://www.stress.org/what_is_stress

7   American Institute of Stress http://www.stress.org/Definition_of_stress.htm

8   http://www.heartmath.com/emwave_technology

9   BREUS, Michael Sleep Habits: More Important Than You Think Chronic Sleep Deprivation May Harm Health http://www.webmd.com/sleep_disorders/features/important_sleep_habits

10 Insufficient sleep is a public health epidemic. http://www.cdc.gove/features/dssleep

11 The Diagnosis and Management of InsomniaJ. Christian Gillin, M.D., and William F. Byerley, M.D.N Engl J Med 1990; 322:239_248January 25, 1990DOI: 10.1056/NEJM199001253220406

12 http://sleepfoundation.org/sleep_tools_tips/healthy_sleep_tips

13 http://sleepfoundation.org/sleep_topics/teens_and_sleep

14 http://www.pursuit_of_happiness.org/history_of_happiness/martin_seligman_positive_psychology/

15 Martin Seligman. Learned Optimism: How to Change Your Mind and Your Life. Vintage Reprint edition 2006

16 Wilhelm, R.(Translator), C. G. Jung (Commentary). The Secret of the Golden Flower: A Chinese Book of Life 1962. A Helen and Kurt Wolff Book

17 Siegel, Bernie. *Love, Medicine & Miracles: Lessons Learned about Self-Healing from a Surgeon's Experience with Exceptional Patients.* Quill, January 1986

18 http://berniesiegelmd.com/products_page/books/

CHAPTER 4 REFERENCES

1 http://www.ncbi.nlm.nih.gov/pmc/articles/PMC2842539/

2 Gbenga O. Ogedegbe, MD; et al. A Randomized Controlled Trial of Positive-Affect Intervention and Medication Adherence in Hypertensive African Americans. JAMA 172(4): 322-326, Feb. 27, 2012. *Arch Intern Med.* 2012;172(4):322-326. doi:10.1001/archinternmed.2011.1307.

3 Hawkes, A.L. et al. Outcomes of coronary artery bypass graft surgery. Vasc Health Risk Manag. Dec 2006; 2(4): 477–484.

4 Tully, PJ. et al. Depression, anxiety, and cardiac morbidity outcomes after coronary artery bypass surgery: a contemporary and practical review. J Geriatr Cardiol. Jun 2012; 9(2): 197–208.

5 DL Katz. Effective dietary counseling: helping patients find and follow "the way" to eat. West Virginia Medical Journal 98(6):256-9, 2002 Nov-Dec

6 Ornish D et al. Lifestyle Heart Trial— Intensive Lifestyle Changes for Reversal of Coronary Heart Disease. *JAMA 280 (23):* 2001-2007, December 16, 1998.

7 http://ornishspectrum.com/undo-it/

8 Stewart, M. et al. The Impact of Patient-Centered Careon Outcomes. The Journal of Family Practice 49(9):796-804, 2000.

9 Beach, M.C. et al. Is the Quality of the Patient-Provider Relationship Associated with Better Adherence and Health Outcomes for Patients with HIV? *J Gen Intern Med.* Jun 2006; 21(6): 661–665.doi: 10.1111/j.1525-1497.2006.00399.x

10 Brenna, N. et al. Trust in the health-care provider–patient relationship: a systematic mapping review of the evidence base. *International Journal for Quality in Health Care 2013: 1-7.* DOI: http://dx.doi.org/10.1093/intqhc/mzt063 First published online: 25 September 2013

11 Stewart, M. et al. The Impact of Patient-Centered Careon Outcomes. TheJournal of Family Practice 49(9):796-804, 2000

12 Walach, H. and Jonas WB. Placebo research: the evidence base for harnessing self-healing capacities. *Altern Complement Med.* 2004;10 Suppl 1:S103-12.

13 Moerman, DE and Jonas, W. Deconstructing the Placebo Effect and Finding the Meaning Response. *Ann Intern Med.* 2002;136(6):471-476. doi:10.7326/0003-4819-136-6-200203190-00011

14 Miller FG, Colloca L and Kaptchuk, T. The placebo effect: illness and interpersonal healing. Perspect Biol Med. 2009 Autumn;52(4):518-39. doi: 10.1353/pbm.0.0115.

15 MK Marvel et al. Soliciting the patient's agenda: have we improved?*JAMA* 281(3): 283-7. 1999

16 Roni Caryn Rabin.(2014)You're on the clock: Doctors rush patients out the door. Kaiser Healt. News.http://www.usatoday.com/story/news/nation/2014/04/20/doctor_visits_time_crunch_health_care/7822161/

17 SHANNON BROWNLEE. Why Your Doctor Has No Time to See You. Newsweek April 16, 2012. http://www.newsweek.com/why_your_doctor_has_no_time_see_you_63949

18 http://www.mymovingreviews.com/move/how_often_and_why_americans_move

19 E. Rosenthal. The Health Care Waiting Game. *The New York Times Sunday Review* July 2014 http://www.nytimes.com/2014/07/06/sunday_review/long_waits_for_doctors_appointments_have_become_the_norm.html?_r=0

20 http://www.nytimes.com/interactive/2014/07/06/sunday_review/waiting_and_waiting.html

21 What bugs you most about your doctor? *Consumer Reports magazine:* June 2013. http://www.consumerreports.org/cro/magazine/2013/06/what_bugs_you_most_about_your_doctor/index.htm

22 Shannon Brownlee. Why Your Doctor Has No Time to See You. Newsweek April 16, 2012. http://www.newsweek.com/why_your_doctor_has_no_time_see_you_63949

23 http://www.cdc.gov/mmwr/preview/mmwrhtml/00042446.htm

24 http://www.schoolwellnesspolicies.org/WellnessPolicies.html

25 National Assoc. of State Boards of Education: State health policy. http://www.nasbe.org/healthy_schools/hs/bytopics.php?topicid=1100

26 California _ Project Lean. http://www.californiaprojectlean.org

27 http://gardens.slowfoodusa.org

28 http://edibleschoolyard.org/network

29 http://www.farmtoschool.org/news_and_articles/looking_back_and_looking_forward_farm_to_school_policy_in_2014_and_2015

30 Personal communication Heather Taffet Gold PhD, Associate Professor, Dept. of Population Health, NYU Medical School.

31 http://www.health.gov/communication/literacy/quickguide/factsbasic.htm

32 Clarke, TC et al. Trends in the Use of Complementary Health Approaches Among Adults: United States, 2002–2012. *National Health Statistics Report Number 79 February 10, 2015*

33 http://altmedicine.about.com/od/alternativemedicinebasics/a/Insurance.htm

APPENDIX 1 REFERENCES

1 http://www.cdc.gov/chronicdisease/overview/index.htm

2 http://www.cdc.gov/chronicdisease/

3 http://www.cdc.gov/chronicdisease/overview/index.htm

4 10 FAQs: Medicare's Role in End-of-Life Carehttp://kff.org/medicare/fact-sheet/10-faqs-medicares-role-in-end-of-life-care/Oct 01, 2015

References

5   David L. Katz, MD, in an Apr. 22, 2014 interview with *Yale Daily News*, "Obesity 'Disease' Discourages Prevention" available at www.yaledailynews.com

6   http://www.ama-assn.org/ama/pub/news/news/2013/2013-06-18-new-ama-policies-annual-meeting.page

7   Centers for Disease Control and Prevention. Exercise or Physical Activity. NCHS FastStats Web site. http://www.cdc.gov/nchs/fastats/exercise.htm. Accessed December 20, 2013.

8   Centers for Disease Control and Prevention. Exercise or Physical Activity. NCHS FastStats Web site. http://www.cdc.gov/nchs/fastats/exercise.htm.

9   Healthy Lifestyles Reduce the Incidence of Chronic Diseases and Dementia: Evidence from the Caerphilly Cohort Study dec 9, 2013 DOI: 10.1371/journal.pone.0081877

10 US Department of Health and Human Services. *The Health Consequences of Smoking—50 Years of Progress: A Report of the Surgeon General.* Atlanta, GA: US Dept of Health and Human Services, Centers for Disease Control and Prevention; 2014

11 Centers for Disease Control and Prevention. Alcohol and Public Health: Alcohol Related Disease Impact (ARDI) Web site. http://apps.nccd.cdc.gov/DACH_ARDI/Default/Default.aspx. Accessed March 11, 2014.

12 Healthy Lifestyles Reduce the Incidence of Chronic Diseases and Dementia: Evidence from the Caerphilly Cohort Study dec 9, 2013 DOI: 10.1371/journal.pone.0081877

13 Heart disease - http://www.cdc.gov/heartdisease/facts.htm

14 Cancer - https://nccd.cdc.gov/uscs/

15 http://www.cancer.org/research/cancerfactsstatistics/cancerfactsfigures2015/index

16 Diabetes - http://www.cdc.gov//diabetes/pubs/statsreport14/national-diabetes-report-web.pdf

17 Obesity, adults - http://www.cdc.gov/obesity/data/adult.html

18 Obesity, childhood - http://www.cdc.gov/obesity/data/childhood.html

19 The State of Obesity 2015. Better Policies for a Healthier America http://healthyamericans.org/reports/stateofobesity2015/

Made in the USA
Columbia, SC
16 December 2017